Pae

We dedicate this book to Professor Dick Smithells,
our mentor, colleague and good friend

Paediatrics

SIR ROY MEADOW
FRCPCH

Emeritus Professor of Paediatrics and Child Health
University of Leeds

SIMON J. NEWELL
FRCPCH

Consultant and Senior Clinical Lecturer in
  Paediatrics and Child Health
St James's University Hospital
Leeds

Seventh Edition

Blackwell
Science

© 2002 by
Blackwell Science Ltd
Editorial Offices:
Osney Mead, Oxford OX2 0EL
25 John Street, London WC1N 2BS
23 Ainslie Place, Edinburgh EH3 6AJ
350 Main Street, Malden
  MA 02148-5018, USA
54 University Street, Carlton
  Victoria 3053, Australia

Other Editorial Offices:
Blackwell Wissenschafts-Verlag GmbH
Kurfürstendamm 57
10707 Berlin, Germany

Blackwell Science KK
MG Kodenmacho Building
7–10 Kodenmacho Nihombashi
Chuo-ku, Tokyo 104, Japan

Iowa State University Press
A Blackwell Science Company
2121 S. State Avenue
Ames, Iowa 50014-8300, USA

First published 1973
Second edition 1975
Third edition 1978
Fourth edition 1981
Fifth edition 1986
Sixth edition 1991
Seventh edition 2002
Reprinted 2002

Set by Best-set Typesetter Ltd., Hong Kong
Printed and bound in Great Britain by
MPG Books Ltd, Bodmin, Cornwall

The Blackwell Science logo is a
trade mark of Blackwell Science Ltd,
registered at the United Kingdom
Trade Marks Registry

DISTRIBUTORS

  Marston Book Services Ltd
  PO Box 269
  Abingdon, Oxon OX14 4YN
  (Orders: Tel: 01235 465500
         Fax: 01235 465555)

The Americas
  Blackwell Publishing
  c/o AIDC
  PO Box 20
  50 Winter Sport Lane
  Williston, VT 05495-0020
  (Orders: Tel: 800 216 2522
          Fax: 802 864 7626)

Australia
  Blackwell Science Pty Ltd
  54 University Street
  Carlton, Victoria 3053
  (Orders: Tel: 3 9347 0300
          Fax: 3 9347 5001)

A catalogue record for this title
is available from the British Library

ISBN 0-632-05065-9

Library of Congress
Cataloging-in-Publication Data

Meadow, R.
    Lecture notes on paediatrics / Roy Meadow,
  Simon J. Newell. — 7th ed.
      p.   cm.
    Includes bibliographical references.
    ISBN 0-632-05065-9 (pbk.)
    1. Pediatrics. I. Newell, Simon J. II. Title.
  RJ45.M43 2001
  618.92 — dc21   2001035386

For further information on
Blackwell Science, visit our
website:
www.blackwell-science.com

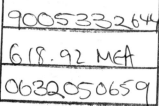

Contents

OSCE Stations

Preface

The first edition of *Lecture Notes on Paediatrics* appeared nearly 30 years ago. Its popularity led to a succession of editions, each of which tended to be rather larger and more detailed than its predecessor (a trend that owed more to the enthusiasm of the authors than the needs of students). Now we return to the original aim of a book containing the necessary factual framework, without the detail that is superfluous for a medical student. The content and the presentation have been refashioned. The inclusion of information boxes and teaching points supplements, rather than replaces, clear text. Objective Structured Clinical Examinations (OSCE) are now used widely in student assessment. An important addition is the inclusion of characteristic OSCE Stations at the end of appropriate chapters to help those who take OSCE exams, and to indicate a sensible approach to common problems.

The re-written chapters and the new sections mean that this edition presents a major change from its predecessors. But the aims defined in the preface to the first edition remain:
'a small book:
• intended to live in the pocket of a white coat, rather than on a bookshelf
• describing the pattern of childhood growth and development, and conditions that are either common, important or interesting. This factual frame work is set against the changing pattern of paediatric practice, the services available for children and the needs of society
• containing sufficient paediatric knowledge for the medical student during the paediatric appointment; but it must be grafted on to preliminary experience of adult medicine and surgery
• with more emphasis on diagnosis than on treatment; therapeutic details are best learned by caring for sick children'.

Professor Dick Smithells and I worked together on six editions, many reprintings, and several translations of *Lecture Notes on Paediatrics*. It was a happy and instructive venture for us both, and it is appropriate that Professor Smithell's place is now taken by someone who was once his student and house officer. Simon Newell is a paediatrician with specialist interest in neonatology and gastroenterology, but above all he is a vigorous and committed teacher, who has a clear vision of the needs of children and their doctors.

Roy Meadow

Acknowledgements

We thank all our colleagues who have helped us over the last 28 years since the publication of the first edition.

The neonatal and cardiovascular chapters are based on the original contributions of Dr Peter Dear and Dr Olive Scott; Dr Adam Craig has made major improvements to the chapter on neoplastic disease; and all the chapters owe much to the original co-author Professor Dick Smithells.

We are indebted to our assistants Mandy Jones and Janet Thompson for their efficient and intelligent work with the manuscripts.

Roy Meadow
Simon Newell

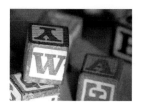

Children and their Health

Children under the age of 16 comprise 20% of the population of the UK and of most industrialized countries, but in many developing countries children represent more than 50% of the population. In all countries children provide a high proportion of a doctor's work. Many GPs find that 30% of their consultations are for children, particularly pre-school children (under 5 years). (Medical students in the middle of a 2- or 3-month paediatric attachment may wonder why only 5% of their training should be devoted to children!)

century has resulted more from preventive (public health) measures than from improved treatment; today virtually the entire population of the UK has safe food and water, free immunization and easy access to local health care. Such is not the case in non-industrialized countries.

> **i** In developing countries:
> 20% lack food
> 20% lack safe drinking water
> 33% lack clothing, shelter, education and health services.

Mortality and morbidity

The health of nations has traditionally been measured by mortality. It seems paradoxical, but it is administratively easier to record deaths and their causes than morbidity, which is more difficult to determine, even for the few diseases (mostly infections) which are notifiable by law. Special studies are needed to determine the incidence of other conditions (Table 1.1).

The causes of death and the patterns of illness in children differ markedly from those in adults. They are influenced by a diversity of factors which include sex, social class, place of birth and season of the year. The decline in child mortality in the past

Child mortality is concentrated in the perinatal period, and the only remaining scope for a *major* reduction in child deaths in the UK lies in better obstetric, neonatal and infant care.

A *stillbirth* refers to a child born dead after the 24th week of pregnancy. A child or fetus born dead earlier in pregnancy is an abortion or miscarriage. A baby that shows signs of life (e.g. heart beat) at birth is a live birth irrespective of the length of gestation.

The continuing fall in UK infant mortality is commendable (Fig. 1.1), but it is salutary to remember that half the countries in the European Union have lower rates. On the other hand, several of the East

UK MORTALITY RATES

Mortality indices	UK rate
Stillbirth rate (Stillbirths per 1000 total births)	5
Early neonatal mortality rate (Deaths in first 7 days per 1000 live births)	3
Perinatal mortality rate (Stillbirths + first week deaths per 1000 total births)	8
Infant mortality rate (Deaths in first year per 1000 live births)	6

Table 1.1 UK mortality rates.

INFANT MORTALITY

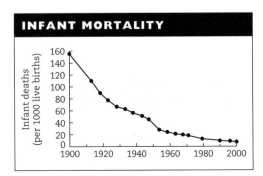

Fig. 1.1 Infant mortality (0–1 years). By 2000, the infant mortality in England and Wales had fallen to a fraction of the level in 1900 (from 156 per 1000 live births to 6 per 1000).

European countries have infant mortality rates 2–3 times higher, and some of the non-industrialized countries would need to be on a different scale altogether. The improvement in infant mortality in the UK has been attributable to the reduction in neonatal mortality; postneonatal mortality (from 1 month to 1 year) shows less improvement. Although some of these deaths result from persistent, serious congenital abnormalities and perinatal problems, and others are the results of accidents or diagnosable disorders, many are infants who die at home, for whom no cause of death is found at autopsy (sudden infant death syndrome, p. 240).

Deaths are concentrated in early life and are higher for boys at all ages, by a factor of 1.3 in the first month of life and by 1.6 for children of school age. For a schoolchild, death is more likely to be due to an accident, particularly a road accident with the child as pedestrian or cyclist, than to any disease. The decline in mortality from infectious diseases has made other serious disorders appear more common. Death from malignancy is now as common as from infection (Figs 1.2 and 1.3).

The pattern of morbidity in children is very different from that of adults (Fig. 1.4). Infections are common, especially of the respiratory, gastrointestinal and urinary tracts, as well as the acute exanthemata. Although degenerative disorders and cerebral vascular accidents are very rare in childhood, new forms of chronic disease are becoming relatively more important as formerly fatal childhood disorders become treatable but not necessarily curable. Thus children with complex congenital heart disease, malignant disease, cystic fibrosis and renal failure receive treatments that all too often leave the child handicapped, either by incomplete cure or the need to live with the difficulties and side-effects of complicated treatment.

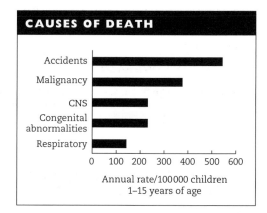

Fig. 1.2 Causes of death in children aged 1–15 years.

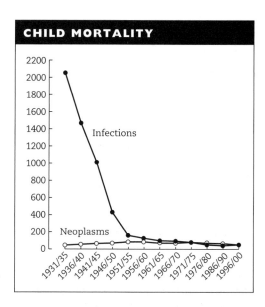

Fig. 1.3 Child mortality from infections and neoplasms, per million children living (aged 1–4 years).

The hallmarks of childhood are growth and development, which influence both the kinds and the patterns of childhood illness. Congenital malformations, genetic disease and the consequences of problems in the perinatal period (e.g. cerebral palsy) are common. Disturbances of development and behaviour, as well as anxiety about normal variants, may demand a lot of the doctor's time.

It has been estimated that a British GP with an average practice would see a new case of pyloric stenosis every 4 years, childhood diabetes every 6 years, Down's syndrome every 16 years, Turner's syndrome every 60 years and haemophilia or Hirschsprung's disease every 600 years! Hospitals may give a very false impression of the pattern of illness in the community at large.

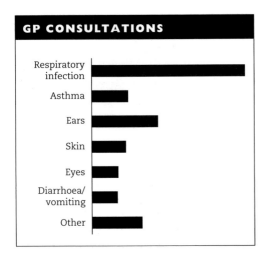

GP CONSULTATIONS

Respiratory infection

Asthma

Ears

Skin

Eyes

Diarrhoea/ vomiting

Other

Fig. 1.4 Commonest reason for a child to be seen by their GP.

Children in society

The Registrar-General's five-point grading of *social class* is a crude but useful classification. Although it depends on the occupation of the father, we recognize that the father's occupation has close correlation with many other important factors including income, housing and attitudes to child rearing.

SOCIOECONOMIC CLASS

I	Higher professional (usually university graduates).
II	Other professional and technical
III	Other non-manual and skilled manual
IV	Semi-skilled manual
V	Unskilled manual

Nearly 10% of children cannot be classified because they do not have a parent with skills or employment. That 'other' category constitutes a group which consistently fares less well than social class V.

The health and educational progress of a child is directly related to the home and the environment. The child of an unskilled worker (social class V) has a 50% greater chance of being born dead or with a serious physical handicap than a lawyer's child (social class I). The disadvantage is there at birth and continues throughout childhood. The social class IV or V child will have more accidents, more physical illnesses, will be smaller and will read less well than the child from social class I or II. Death rates for younger children are more than twice as high as those of older children. At any age a child from social class V is twice as likely to die as one from social class I (Table 1.2).

This class difference has remained much the same, or even widened, over the last 30 years despite overall improvements in mortality and morbidity rates. Family size and birth order can also be important; the later children of large families tend to be smaller and have an increased chance of death in infancy or handicap later on.

The proportion of children born outside marriage has risen to nearly 40% of all births. Over half of the children born outside marriage have parents who are living together, and are therefore likely to be brought up within a stable home. One-third are born to women under the age of 20 and many of those children stay with their

Table 1.2 Social class and childhood mortality: death rates per 100 000.

CHILDHOOD MORTALITY					
	Social class				
Age	I	II	III	IV	V
1–4	33	34	46	64	116
5–9	24	19	24	31	45
10–14	20	22	23	31	36

mother or grandmother in what is often an unsatisfactory home. The change in the traditional pattern of family life and the increase in marital breakdown (one in three marriages ends in divorce) have resulted in about 15% of all families with children being single-parent families.

> **Government objective:**
> To reduce the rate of conception among those under 16 to < 4.8/1000.

Unsatisfactory homes are not just those where there is overt cruelty, poverty or squalor. Stress at home may result from parental discord — quarrelling and separations, one-parent families, and children who have been put in the care of an unsuitable parent after divorce. It may result from parental illness — a dying or chronically handicapped mother, a mentally ill father, or just from parental inadequacy (work-shy or drunken parents and those who have abandoned the struggle of trying to be satisfactory parents).

The doctor sees the childhood casualties of these social events: poor development, illness and behavioural problems. Teachers see the casualties, too: unhappy children, delinquent children and children whose school progress is inappropriately slow.

The complexity and multiplicity of the factors that cause a child to be disadvantaged sometimes makes us feel helpless. However, since adversities compound one another, much may be achieved by modifying even one adverse factor. Even if we feel discouraged, it is worth trying to modify some aspects of the child's life to try to achieve at least one of the following factors:
- self-esteem (we need to feel wanted)
- one good human relationship (we need to feel trusted)
- firm supervision and discipline (we need rules).

Extensive medical and social services exist, particularly for handicapped children, but all too often they are best used by well-informed, middle-class parents, while the parents of the disadvantaged child do not use them sometimes because they do not know about them. All medical and paramedical staff have a duty to recognize children in need or in distress and to see that they benefit from the help that is available.

> **i** Twenty percent of the world's population live in absolute poverty. Nearly half of them are children.

Community medical services

Community paediatrician

Most paediatricians have a commitment to some services outside of the hospital. Community paediatricians specialize in working outside of the hospital, and usually have a limited role within it. Many of them are responsible for child health surveillance and children's services in a specific geographical sector. Others specialize in particular areas of work—learning problems, child protection (child abuse), or audiology. They work closely with health visitors and the staff of child health clinics, and also with GPs, social and educational services.

Health visitors

These are registered nurses with additional training in preventative health care. Many are attached to general practices and a few specialize (e.g. in diabetes) and have hospital attachments. They are responsible for family health, and particularly for mothers and young children. Their job is to prevent illness and handicap by giving appropriate advice, by detecting problems early and by mobilizing services to deal with those problems. They have an important role in child health promotion.

Child health clinics

These clinics should be readily accessible to mothers with young children, and may be located in health centres, village halls or in purpose-built accommodation. They are staffed by health visitors and doctors and play an important role in child health surveillance, offering routine medical and developmental examinations for infants and pre-school children, immunization, health education, and advice and support for those with special problems. About 90% of babies attend such a clinic during their first year, but thereafter attendance falls off.

Parent-held Child Health Record

Parents should be encouraged to take the 'red book' whenever the child attends clinic or hospital. It contains a permanent record of child health surveillance, the child's growth including a centile chart, hospital visits, health education and advice. When seeing a child a doctor should ask

to see the book and thank the parent for having it readily available.

Child health surveillance

Child health promotion focuses on both primary and secondary prevention of problems. *Child health surveillance* is part of the programme and refers specifically to secondary prevention by means of the early detection of existing problems.

The programme of surveillance is a combined undertaking, starting at birth with the hospital doctor or midwife and then involving the primary health care team: health visitor, GP and then the school health service. As the Department of Health points out, it cannot start too early, for 'every effort should be made to ensure that women of child bearing age are themselves healthy and that, by sensible family planning, pregnancies are welcome'.

Immunization

See p. 218.

Health education and preparation for parenthood

During the final years at school and in the antenatal period, there are numerous opportunities for health education and training in *parentcraft*. The following information contributes to reduction of child mortality and morbidity:

- the dangers of delaying antenatal care
- the importance of good nutrition
- the adverse effects of smoking and alcohol during pregnancy
- the importance of love, care, nurture and play
- the importance of breast feeding: bottle feeding techniques
- parental smoking and respiratory disease in children
- how to recognize when a child is ill

CHILD HEALTH SURVEILLANCE

Monitoring development

- Programme schedule
  - At birth, clinical examination (p. 58) (doctor or midwife).
  - 6–10 days. Full clinical examination (GP).
  - 6 weeks. Assessment of well-being, weight gain and development (GP/health visitor).
  - 7–8 months. Review of development. Screening tests for vision and hearing (GP/health visitor).
  - 18–24 months. Review of development, especially social and language (health visitor in the home). Opportunity to discuss toilet training.
  - 3–3$\frac{1}{2}$ years. General review including hearing, vision, squint, teeth. Opportunity to discuss emotional and social problems.
  - 5 years. School entry—general medical check during first school year (school nurse/doctor).
  - School years. Regular checks of growth, hearing, vision, teeth. Testing of colour vision (especially boys) at 8–9 years. Examination of children about whom parents or teachers are concerned. Opportunities for older children to refer themselves to school doctor or nurse.

- Screening tests
  - Phenylketonuria and hypothyroidism at 4–8 days.
  - Congenital dislocation of the hip—at birth; 6–10 days; 6 weeks.
  - Hearing and vision as above.

- how to minimize the risks of accidents at home and on the road
- the importance of dental health
- the role of the father.

> Government objective:
> A reduction in smoking in pregnancy of at least one-third.

School health service

The school health service was established in 1904 because 40% of young men volunteering for service in the Boer War were found to be medically unfit. Today its main functions are to assess the state of health of schoolchildren, to help with the educational problems created by ill health and to promote better health. The service is particularly important for children from unsatisfactory homes who may have missed pre-school health checks.

School nurses are responsible, in conjunction with teachers, for identifying schoolchildren with disorders that are likely to interfere with their development, education and happiness, and for ensuring that they are seen by the community paediatrician.

Nursery schools

These may be separate schools or nursery classes attached to primary schools. They cater for children aged 3–5 years and are staffed by teachers specially trained in child development working with *nursery nurses* and assistants. They aim to encourage a child's development and learning by play, stimulation and physical activity.

Day nurseries

These cater for two main groups of pre-school children: those who require daytime care whilst their parents are at work or ill (particularly those who only have a single parent) and children from disadvantaged homes. They are staffed by trained nursery nurses. The number of day nurseries is few and the demand is large, which has led to groups of parents forming their own centres for pre-school children, variously named play groups, play centres or crèches.

INCIDENCE OF SOME IMPORTANT PROBLEMS

At 1 year:
- 10% of boys have been circumcised

At 5 years:
- 7% have had at least one seizure
- 5% have a squint
- 5% have a behavioural problem
- 5% have a speech or language problem
- 2% have a substantial congenital defect

At 7 years:
- 15% have eczema, asthma or hay fever
- 13% require special education
- 10% wet their beds
- 2% have had a hernia repair
- <1% have had an appendicectomy

Social services

The social services department of the local authority is responsible for the care and/or supervision of children up to 18 years in a variety of circumstances: if they cannot be cared for by their parents, by reason of their illness or death, or because the children have been abandoned or lost. The local authority may be designated a 'fit person' to assume parental rights in order to provide security and protection for the child. Parental rights may be given to the local authority by the Court (usually a Family or Juvenile Court), in which case a child is said to be the subject of a *care order*. The Court must be satisfied that the child has suffered, or is likely to suffer, significant harm because of the standard of parental care or because of being beyond parental control. 'Harm' includes ill-treatment, sexual abuse, and the impairment of good physical and mental health and development.

The local authority tries to keep or place children with their own parents, relatives or friends. When this is not possible, the child is looked after by the local authority in:

Foster homes (65%) in which a child is cared for in a family other than his own. Brief placements are successful, but long-term fostering less so. There are an increasing number of schemes in which the foster parents are paid extra to look after children with physical and mental handicap or disturbed adolescents.

Residential placements: Children's Homes, Residential Schools and Secure Units (35%) aim to provide as normal an upbringing as possible, despite frequent changes of staff. They contain a higher proportion of difficult or handicapped children than foster homes. Of children in these homes, 95% still have a living parent, so that many are visited regularly or may be reunited with their parents for weekends or longer periods.

Children may be supervised in their own homes, either on a voluntary basis or as a result of a court *supervision order*. The social worker's prime aim is to prevent family break-up and to help with problems of care, physical and emotional. He or she works as part of a team with others involved with the family, e.g. health visitors, doctors, teachers.

CHILDREN ACT 1989

The Act affects all aspects of the welfare and protection of children including day-care, fostering and adoption, child abuse and the consequences for children of marital breakdown. The spirit of the Act is reflected in the opening paragraphs:

'the child's' welfare shall be the court's paramount consideration'.

'any delay in determining the question (of the child's upbringing) is likely to prejudice the welfare of the child'.

'a court shall have regard to . . . the ascertainable wishes and feelings of the child concerned'.

If the parents are married at the time of the child's birth, both have parental responsibilities. If they were not married, the mother has parental responsibility, but there are legal mechanisms by which the father can acquire it.

The social services department is responsible for supervising children placed privately with foster parents. People who look after other people's children, whether on a day (child day-care, childminder) or residential (foster) basis, must register with their local social services department, even though they may be paid direct by the parent.

Social Services also provide advice about financial benefits available from the Departments of Social Security. In relation to children, the mobility component of the *Disability Living Allowance* (DLA) is available from the age of 5 years; a care component for infants requiring specially close supervision or attention to bodily functions is available from birth.

Voluntary services

The statutory services are supplemented by a large number of voluntary and charitable organizations, many of which were in existence before, and paved the way for, statutory provisions. Many of those offering services to children have a high level of professional expertise. The NSPCC (National Society for the Prevention of Cruelty to Children) and its Scottish counterpart continue their historic role of protecting children, and giving advice and support to families under stress. Barnardo's, the Children's Society and the National Children's Homes have adapted their activities to the changing pattern of child needs. The Save the Children Fund gives support to deprived inner cities in the UK as well as relief in developing countries. Many voluntary bodies receive some funding from central and/or local government.

Parent support groups exist for almost every chronic disorder of childhood (e.g. Cystic Fibrosis Trust). Their membership consists largely of parents of affected children who can offer advice to others from first-hand experience. They also raise money to support research, thereby augmenting the work of the major medical research charities.

The *Family Fund* exists to give financial help to less well-off families with very severely handicapped children. It is financed by the Department of Health, but administered by the Rowntree Trust in York. Charitable organizations can often minimize bureaucracy and cut administrative costs and delays.

Adoption

Couples wishing to adopt a child approach either their local authority or a registered adoption society. Each agency tends to have its own requirements, for instance attachment to a particular religious denomination, or an age limit — it is difficult to adopt a child if you are over 40. The agencies' main concern will be relationships within the family, but it is also important for applicants to have a steady income, a settled home and satisfactory health. Once accepted the applicants have to wait anything from a few months to several years, until a suitable child is placed with them. The child is now a full member of the adoptive family; he or she takes their name and has all the rights of a natural child (except that he or she cannot inherit a title!).

Medical examinations are required for both parents, for the child before placement and again before the adoption order is made in court. It is essential to explain and discuss any suspected handicaps with the prospective parents. Parents are also advised to inform their child from the beginning that they are adopted and to explain this regularly and more fully as the child's understanding increases.

Adoptive parents are carefully selected, therefore adoptive children with a history of severe deprivation or abuse tend to fare rather better than they would have done in their natural family.

Children in hospital

Until the middle of the nineteenth century the training of doctors and the provision of medical services, including hospitals, did not recognize the particular needs of children. In the following decades, when people like Charles Dickens and Lord Shaftesbury were stirring the public conscience to recognize the appalling circumstances in which many children grew up (or failed to do so), children's hospitals were established. The birth and development of paediatrics as a medical specialty was largely attributable to these hospitals, and

they gave excellent service for a century or more.

In the later decades of the twentieth century, the pattern of hospital care for children changed. Children still have special needs — unrestricted visiting, facilities for resident mothers, play activities for younger children, education for older children — but the children's ward of today differs greatly from that of 40 years ago:
• child in-patients are, on average, much younger
• they are more severely ill
• they need greater facilities for investigation and treatment
• the average stay in hospital is much shorter
• parents are actively involved in care
• many medical and surgical procedures are done as day-cases
• neonatal care makes increasingly heavy demands on resources.
Although the number of children admitted to hospital has increased as new therapies have become available, their shorter stay in hospital means that fewer children's beds are needed. This, coupled with the need for access to expensive investigational technology, has resulted in the closure of most children's hospitals and the establishment of children's units in general hospitals (Fig. 1.5).

Hospitals are not without risk to patients, especially child patients. The hazard of cross-infection is obvious: the hazard of mother–child separation is less obvious but can be more serious, especially among the 1–4 year olds. At this age children are old enough to grieve for a lost mother, but not old enough to understand the reason, or that the separation is temporary. 'Tomorrow' has no meaning for a toddler.

A young child separated from the mother may go through three stages:
Protest: he cries for her return.
Withdrawal: he curls up with a comfort

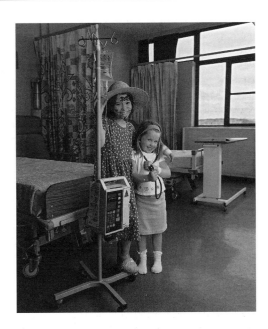

Fig. 1.5 Children in hospital.

blanket or toy and loses interest in food and play.

Denial: he appears happy, making indiscriminate friendships with everybody. This can be mistakenly interpreted as the child having 'settled', but the mother–child bond has been damaged and will have to be rebuilt. On returning home he may exhibit tantrums, refuse food or wet his bed.

These problems can be avoided or minimized by:

• avoiding hospital admission if possible
• reducing the length of any admission to the minimum
• performing operations (e.g. herniotomy, orchidopexy) and investigations (e.g. jejunal biopsy, colonoscopy) as day cases
• encouraging parents to visit often and arranging for one to sleep alongside a young child.

Hospital organization can also help to reduce stress. Children should be grouped together so that they may be looked after by staff specially trained and experienced in the care of children. Registered general nurses usually see little of children during their training and need further experience if they are to hold senior posts on children's units; the same is true of therapists. Teachers, nursery nurses and play leaders organize education and play. Segregation from adults allows children's wards to be less formal. The first impression of a children's ward should be of happy chaos, rather than of the highly technical medicine which is in fact going on.

Immigrant families

The history of most countries involves the assimilation of new cultures and people from other lands, for man has always been a great traveller. Assimilation is usually gradual and in the early years beset with problems. Most countries today have immigrant communities with particular needs. In the UK, 5% of the population (and nearly 10% of the newborn) are of Asian or West Indian origin. Those figures disguise great regional variations from areas almost devoid of new commonwealth immigrants to others, such as Bradford, where 30% of the newborn are of Pakistani origin.

ETHNIC COMPOSITION— ENGLAND AND WALES

White	94%
Indian continent	3%
Black	2%
Other	1%

In general, particular sects of immigrants tend to live together, so that certain towns and cities may have a preponderance of one or other sect (e.g. Gujarati Indians in Leicester). It is worth finding out if local immigrants are mainly of a particular sect or religion and being aware of some of the differences.

The main medical problems and misunderstandings occur in relation to the large groups from the Indian subcontinent.
• North-east Pakistan and Bangladesh, usually *Muslim* (Islamic religion).
• Gujarat in north-west India, mainly *Hindu*.
• Punjab in northern India, usually *Sikh*.

There are several important medical aspects:

Names
Selecting the appropriate and polite name can be difficult. Sikh boys have the complementary name Singh, and girls Kaur. The personal name precedes the complementary name and the subcaste name (surname) follows it, e.g. Davindar Kaur Bhumbra. The Hindu naming system is somewhat similar. Devi for girls and Lal for boys are common complementary names, and may be joined on to the first personal name, e.g. Arima Devi Chopra becomes Arimadevi Chopra. Some Sikhs and Hindus will not use a subcaste name. Muslim names

are more difficult; often there is no shared family name. Males have a religious title (e.g. Mohammed or Abdul) which may precede or follow the personal name. Females have a title (e.g. Begum or Bibi) and a personal name. It is discourteous to use the religious name or title on its own: it must be coupled with the personal name. (In close friendship the personal name is used on its own without the religious name or title.)

Contact with foreign diseases
Most children will have been born and brought up in Britain. But if the child has recently arrived in the country, or returned from visiting relatives in the parents' homeland, he or she is at risk of unusual illnesses (malaria is seen in children returning from Pakistan and hookworm in those from tropical and subtropical regions) and diseases that are more common abroad (e.g. tuberculosis in India and Pakistan).

Racial susceptibility to disease
Some diseases are exclusive to certain races, e.g. sickle-cell disease in blacks. More commonly a disease is simply more likely in particular races, e.g. thalassaemia major in Pakistanis and Cypriots. The indigenous white British person is more likely to be born with cystic fibrosis or spina bifida, and is particularly susceptible to refractive errors—spectacles are part of the national uniform for the over forties. *Consanguinity* (marrying a blood relative) is common in some cultures, particularly among Muslims. The offspring have an increased chance of receiving the same recessive gene from each parent, and of developing an otherwise rare genetically determined disease.

Food
Asian families are prone to nutritional problems because of the difficult compromise they have to achieve between their religious beliefs and the food industry.

Orthodox Hindus are vegetarian, less strict Hindus avoid beef. Muslims avoid pork, and any meat must be killed in a special way (Halal). Muslim children at puberty may join *Ramadan*, the month-long fast, each year.

Customs

Asian women avoid exposure to sunlight: vitamin D deficiency is common in pregnancy and is a risk for their newborn babies. As the girls reach puberty they adopt traditional clothes which shield their limbs and skin from sunlight; the chance of rickets is increased. Orthodox Muslim women are relatively confined to the home, and lead a restricted life; very often the husband will be responsible for all outside activities including taking the child to a doctor or hospital. The person accompanying the child to the clinic may be the most senior male member of the family or the best at speaking English, yet know little of the child's problem or the mother's worries. Parents who themselves were brought up and educated in a developing country may have old-fashioned beliefs about health, and often have no recognition that emotional factors may cause or exacerbate pain.

The cumulative effect of these social and cultural factors is important for the child from conception and through school. Thus the Muslim mother in Britain compared with her white neighbours is more likely to be in social class IV or V, to conceive before the age of 15 or after the age of 35, to have more than four children, to have less antenatal care, more anaemia and a baby of low birth weight. The rates for stillbirth, infant death and major congenital abnormalities are twice as great, and the chance of the child requiring special education even greater. Enquiring about the racial background or the family cultural and religious beliefs should not be a source of embarrassment; nor is it a basis for unfair discrimination. In practice we behave as

if all children are born equal — then we respect and cater for their differences and difficulties. We want an aristocracy of achievement.

Laws relating to the young

For legal purposes a child remains a 'child' up to the age of 14, is a 'young person' up to 17, and is an adult at 18. However, many laws become operative at other ages.

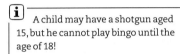 A child may have a shotgun aged 15, but he cannot play bingo until the age of 18!

School education is compulsory for children aged 5 and over. Children may not leave school until they are 16.

Work

Children may not be employed until they are 13. Then they may be employed only between the hours of 7 a.m. and 7 p.m., and for a maximum of 2 h on school days.

ABUSE

It is an offence to:
- tattoo anyone under 18
- seduce a girl under 16
- sell tobacco to a child under 16
- sell fireworks to a child under 13
- expose to fire risk a child under 12
- give intoxicating liquor to children under 5.

Crime

Children under 10 (under 8 in Scotland) are not considered 'criminally responsible' for their misdeeds, and may be dealt with by the Juvenile Courts.

The court can make (1) a *Care Order* giving parental rights to the local authority; or (2) a *Supervision Order* which may be administered by the social services department or, if the child is over 14, by the probation department. At the age of 15 children can be sent to youth custody.

Adult courts deal with those over the age of 17. Although it is legally possible to be sent to prison for a first offence at the age of 17, in practice it is rare before the age of 20.

At the age of 100 the child may receive a telegram of congratulation from the Queen!

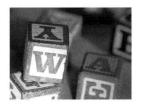

Parents and Children: listening and talking

When compared with other animal species, *Homo sapiens* takes an inordinate length of time to achieve independence from parents. Throughout most of childhood, therefore, parents must act as the child's advocate. Parents tell us about the child's symptoms — although the children contribute more and more as they grow older — and put into effect any treatments needed outside hospital.

Small children only survive because their parents are concerned about them. A few are less concerned than they should be, and their children suffer from neglect. Others are more than usually concerned. Doctors tend to refer to them as anxious or over-anxious and they may be regarded as a nuisance, forever cluttering a busy GP's surgery. These different patterns often reflect the parents' own upbringing, as do excessive concerns with physiological functions, such as eating, sleeping and bowel habits.

Most parents want their children to succeed — to be above average in height and intelligence, to be at least in the top half and preferably in the top 10%. Some parents want their children to succeed in fields that are important to them, such as sport; some want them to help with, and later take over, a family business; most hope that their children will have achievements or material possessions that they did not have themselves.

Paediatric history-taking is therefore complex and often time-consuming. The doctor must try to disentangle the factual account from parental interpretations and overtones (Table 2.1).

History-taking

The child's history covers the same ground as that of an adult patient, with some important additions.

• Address the parents as 'Mr or Mrs Jackson', not as mum or dad.

• Find out what the child is called at home and use that name.

• Begin the history with the name, sex, and the age in years and months (though there is little significant difference between two students aged 21 and 21$\frac{1}{2}$ years, toddlers of 14 and 20 months are quite different). Accurate age is essential and often defines the differential diagnosis.

• Note the name of the school, nursery, clinic or health centre she attends.

• During the history, a young child may be happiest on a parent's knee; a more independent one may prefer playing with toys, which should be available. An older child must be fully included in the discussion. Arrange the furniture to encourage a sense of partnership between parents and doctor and avoid confrontation over the top of a desk.

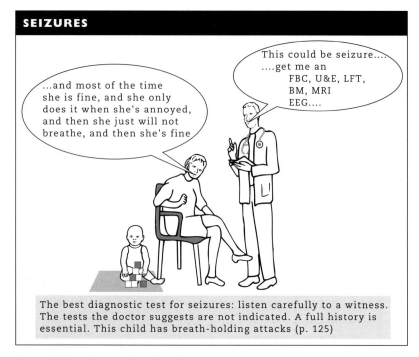

Fig. 2.1 The best diagnostic test for seizures.

FACT	INTERPRETATION
She has vomited three times	Our baby has colic
He has had a rash	He is not eating properly
She gets wheezy when she runs	She was feverish
He falls asleep at school	He is lazy at school

Table 2.1 Fact/interpretation.

If the parents do not speak English, insist upon an interpreter.

History of the presenting condition

Begin with this because it is what they have come to tell you about. Let them tell it their own way first; then ask specific questions to fill in necessary details (Fig. 2.1). Frequent interruptions or insistence on ordered chronology will inhibit free speech. To assess severity, find out how the illness is affecting the child's life. Does the acute asthma stop the child from running, walking, talking; if the problem is not acute, how much school has been missed through illness? School is the equivalent of an adult's employment. Has the child opted out of games or of leisure activities at home? Ask about patterns of eating, sleeping and activity. If these have not changed, serious illness is unlikely. A diminution in appetite or activity, or an increased need for sleep, are likely to be significant. Recorded weight loss is always important.

Ask for the parents' own ideas about what is the matter with the child. Sometimes it will enable you to assuage an unnecessary anxiety; at other times it may lead to a correct diagnosis you had not considered. Mothers are more likely than anyone else to understand their babies' cries, and research shows that babies can 'talk'. They have different cries for hunger, pain, etc. The mother will usually know when the cry is abnormal and sometimes will be able to suggest a reason.

> Listen to the mother — she will tell you the diagnosis.

It is often helpful, especially if psychological problems are suspected, to ask 'What kind of boy (girl) is he (she)? The answer may be 'a worrier', 'placid', 'never still', 'obsessional'. If you then ask 'Who does he take after?', it often provides useful insight for the parent. It is also helpful to know what the child does in his spare time and whether he is by nature gregarious or solitary.

> Make a note of who gave you the history.

Previous medical history
• Illnesses, operations or hospital attendances
• Allergies or drug sensitivities
• Immunization history: it may help to exclude a suspected condition, and it identifies those families in need of advice about further immunization.
• Ask the parents for their child's parent-held health record (and thank them for

having brought it). The booklet includes details of previous weights, immunizations and other health events.

Family history
• The ages of the siblings and parents.
• Whether any other member of the family has, or has had, the same condition as the child, whether it be a rash and fever (has the child caught the same infection?), or six digits on each hand (has the child an inherited condition that runs in the family?).
• What illnesses the parents and close relatives have had, in order to allay needless worries. The parents may worry that their child's stomach ache is caused by stomach cancer, because a relative recently died with it.
• An enquiry regarding consanguinity, especially in Muslim families, because rare inherited conditions are more likely if the parents are related.

> Diagnostic signs on examination are rare; the child's diagnosis lies in the history.

Perinatal history
• Pregnancy gestation (normal is 40 weeks)
  ♦ illnesses
• Delivery place (hospital/home)
  ♦ presentation (head/breech)
  ♦ type (spontaneous, forceps, caesarian section)
  ♦ birth weight
• Neonatal period
  ♦ abnormalities
  ♦ illnesses
  ♦ need for special/intensive care
  ♦ day of discharge home.

Developmental history
This is almost unique to paediatrics. It is important, particularly for young or handicapped children. It includes details of the times at which skills such as walking

and talking were acquired (full details in Chapter 4).

Social history

After establishing rapport with the parents, talk with them about their life, their home, their work and their problems. Find out the father's job (it is a useful financial guide), and find out exactly what the job entails; a 'lorry driver' may be a local parcel deliverer or a long-distance lorry driver who is away from home much of the time. Does the mother go out to work and, if so, who looks after the child? If the mother is now a housewife, what was her job before? If she was a nurse, she will have a different level of knowledge and a different need for information. Three particular areas must be explored which have a direct influence on the child's development:

• The family composition: are the mother and father living together? If so, in harmony or discord? Is this a single-parent family?

• The financial situation: is the family financially viable, or are they dependent on income support?

• Housing: do they have a home of their own, and if so, what sort? Are they living with relatives or in a hostel? Satisfactory housing should have a supply of hot water and indoor sanitation, and not more than 1.5 persons per room.

We each find some parents easy to interview, and others difficult. It is as well to get into the habit of blaming ourselves if the history is unclear. If you are tempted to label someone a 'bad historian', remember that a historian is the person who collects and records the history!

The consultation

When the family arrive they will be waiting anxiously for the doctor's 'verdict'. Their fears are usually far worse than the reality. Talking to the child and parents, explain 'first I would like you to tell me about it, then I will examine Susan, tell you what I think, and we can decide what we want to do about it'. With the history and examination completed, you will probably know enough to point the conversation in one of three directions:

• explanation and reassurance
• investigation and/or treatment but with a favourable outcome probable
• bad news.

Reassurance is readily accepted by some parents who 'just wanted to make sure everything was all right'. An experienced doctor may detect that the child's condition was only a pretext to visit him, and that more serious concerns lie elsewhere. Others are very difficult to reassure. Careful explanation is usually helpful. People rarely stop worrying because somebody says 'Don't worry', but they may stop if they understand why the doctor is not worried. A specific anxiety needs an equally specific reassurance. Thus, if parents fear that their child's pallor may be due to leukaemia, a normal blood count may be insufficient reassurance. They need to hear the doctor say 'She has not got leukaemia'.

Investigations and treatments must be explained in advance to parents and to children old enough to understand. Be honest. Many blood tests require a needle in a vein, and that is painful. A CT scan is noisy (or, for very young children, may require a general anaesthetic). Children are very forgiving if you are honest with them.

Parents want to know the results of tests, and their implications, as soon as possible. Do not keep them waiting unnecessarily. Everyone else uses the telephone — so can doctors.

Treatments to be given by parents must be explained and reasons given (e.g. why four times a day?). Techniques for the use of inhalers for asthma, injections for diabetes or rectally administered anticonvulsants must be demonstrated.

Parents are far more informed about medical matters than were their parents, principally from television, newspapers, magazines, and the internet. Unfortunately the media tend to exaggerate or sensation-alize, presenting an experimental new treatment as a 'breakthrough', or a particu-lar clinic or hospital (often in another coun-try) as 'the only one of its kind' and hence, by implication, the best. The accolade of TV hype is more impressive than holy writ, and the doctor trying to put things in perspec-tive may have an uphill task. We need special understanding for parents who have been offered hope when they had none before.

Bad news usually concerns:
- birth defect in a newborn baby
- a serious handicap in a young child
- a serious, progressive or incurable disease.

The news that a baby is deformed is a great shock to the parents. Even minor anomalies are seen as major tragedies. At the first interview detailed explanations will not be grasped. If the baby is to be transferred to another hospital for surgery, the mother must have a chance to see her infant before transfer and she will need frequent progress reports on the baby until she is able to visit. If the baby survives, the parents need detailed explanation of the care needed and how to recognize any problems that are likely to arise. Parents of children with serious defects or handicaps will need advice about the recurrence risks if they plan another child later on. For easily rec-ognizable conditions in which a genetic (or non-genetic) basis is clearly established, the family doctor or paediatrician can provide this information. For more complex prob-lems reference to a *genetic counselling* clinic is advisable. The three basic essentials for counselling are:

- a firmly established diagnosis, which is often more difficult than it sounds
- a full family history
- ample time to elicit facts and anxieties, and to explain recurrence risks, prenatal tests and other relevant issues.

All this implies ready access to doctors and nurses who can listen and answer, and who can at least give the appearance of having unlimited time to spare. Parents' self help groups can provide information, leaflets and mutual support. Parents should be told about them.

In summary, whenever serious disease is diagnosed in a child parents want to know:
- Exactly what is the matter, in terms they can grasp;
- What the doctors can do about it;
- What the parents can do about it;
- The outlook for this child;
- The outlook for any other children that may follow;
- Why it happened. Did they cause it?

Parents' reactions to bad news tend to follow a recognizable pattern, although the timescale varies widely from one family to another. It is important to recognize this, not only for the purposes of helping, but so that the doctor is not hurt by finding himself the target of parental anger, or irritated by the difficulties of communication.

The stages of adaptation to personal tragedy, which often overlap, are as follows.

1 Intellectual and emotional numbness. In-formation does not get in. Emotions do not get out. The doctor may be relieved that the parents have 'taken it so well'. She may later be annoyed if parents say 'nobody told us anything' when she spent hours telling them everything.

2 Denial. The message has got through but cannot yet be believed. 'There must be some mistake' or 'But he will catch up, won't he?' are characteristic of this stage. The doctor must resist the temptation to hedge or to use woolly phrases such as

'slow developer' which encourage parents to believe that the problem is curable.

3 Guilt and anger. Now the truth has registered and blame must be apportioned. Parents usually blame themselves for some act of commission or omission, real or imaginary. The feeling of guilt may be so intolerable that they need to blame somebody else, personal (the doctor) or impersonal (the tablets).

4 All being well, this is followed by grieving, which is a natural and healing process. Tears are appropriate, and if they are shed in the presence of the doctor he or she should not be embarrassed. They represent a privileged communication and tell the doctor that the final stage is near.

5 Reconstruction. The former pattern of family life has been demolished; the new must now be built. It is imperative that the parents are given a key, active role in any therapeutic programme. Never say 'Nothing can be done'—it is not true (Fig. 2.2).

Involving the child

Children from about 2 years can hear, understand and say a lot. By 7 or 8 years, they are wise. Don't talk about them as if they had no understanding—and you may have to discourage parents from doing the same. Some doctors who commence the consultation talking with parent and child together conclude by talking with each privately—'Please will you wait outside whilst I talk with your mother and then I will ask her to wait outside whilst I talk with you: so that will be fair to everyone'.

As children with chronic illness approach adolescence, parents find it particularly difficult to loosen the apron-strings. The doctor can make a small contribution by treating young teenagers as equal with parents during consultations, and, as they get older, by talking principally with the young patient.

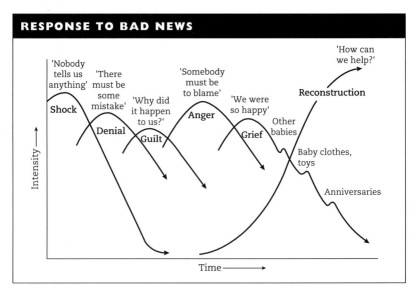

Fig. 2.2 Emotional response to bad news.

By the same token, whatever the medical problem, the child is first a child. Not 'he is a diabetic' or 'she is an epileptic': he has diabetes, she has epilepsy.

Finally, do not, in conversation with parents, refer to their baby as 'it'. If in doubt, better to risk an incorrect 'he' or 'she' than render their infant sexless.

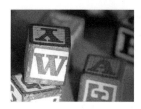

Examination of Children

Examining children, especially the very young, seems daunting to students, but most children are cooperative and clinical examination should be a happy experience for them. Children are usually accompanied by a parent, who will help the doctor and appreciate being involved.

The obvious reason for examination is to find abnormal signs that help make the diagnosis. In acute illness, symptoms are often non-specific, the general impression of a child's health is all important, and essential signs (e.g. infected throat, stiff neck or infected urine) will be missed if the doctor does not look for them systematically. In more protracted illness, specific signs are often absent. The detection of minor congenital abnormalities can be useful.

Parents and children often come to the paediatrician concerned about severe disease. A 'thorough examination' is a powerful therapeutic weapon in the face of parental anxiety. Parents do not readily accept reassurance from the doctor who has not examined the child—and quite right too!

Children of different ages require different approaches.

• Newborn infants: in the early weeks of life, patience, warm hands and a quiet voice are needed. Bedside manner contributes little.

• 2–10 months: infants respond to the friendly doctor, and examination is often easy if the child is generally comfortable. Rapport, and even cooperation, can be found.

• 10 months—2 years: toddlers present the biggest challenge to doctors. The toddler is generally suspicious of strangers. Their confidence must be won, perhaps by giving them something to hold; an unhurried, confident approach is most likely to lead to success. Young children do not like to be separated from their parents, rapidly undressed or made to lie flat. Examining a child on the mother's knee, or standing close beside her, is usually more successful than putting the child on an examination couch. The doctor must be patient and adaptable—the pace and the order of the examination will be dictated by the child.

• 5–10 years: school age children are used to being without their parents, but still want them close by in unfamiliar surroundings. They are generally cooperative. They enjoy neurological examination and like to listen to their heart through a stethoscope. A worried child can be diverted by chatting to them.

• 10 years to teenage: the process of examining the older child and teenager is usually straightforward. Cooperation is almost guaranteed if the doctor respects the child's independence and maturity. Ask them whether they would prefer their parents to be present, and seek their permission to examine them. Often the history taking will be dominated by a parent, and most teenagers cannot tell you their birthweight! The time of the examination is an opportunity to talk to the older child about their complaints.

A system of examination

In acute paediatrics, outpatients, and in undergraduate exams, clinical examination begins with general assessment and then moves on to look at specific systems. All who are new to paediatrics must begin by learning these skills.

> A good history will raise specific questions, e.g. this history could be pneumonia. Is this child unwell? Is she tachypnoeic or febrile?

Initial assessment

Clinical examination has certain essential elements; these are made during the first approach to the child and should be carefully recorded. The most striking finding in a young child with pneumonia, for example, is that they appear ill. The positive clinical findings of lobar consolidation are difficult to elicit, and may be absent.

OSCE stations

Many additional points of importance in clinical assessment are made in the specific chapters. At the end of most chapters is an OSCE station, which offers specific hints and tips which are aimed to help students when they are being assessed. The following is a guide to the OSCE station format. The first OSCE station appears at the end of this chapter.

OBJECTIVE STRUCTURED CLINICAL EXAMINATION (OSCE)

OSCE has now become the most widely used method of assessing clinical skills. The principle is simple. The examiners first determine what is required of the candidate. A simple standardized question is given to the candidate (e.g. please examine this 4-year-old boy's cardiovascular system), and the candidate is observed by the examiner, who ticks off essential elements of examination technique. Further marks are given for general approach, rapport with the child and their parent, and interpretation of the findings.

In the OSCE examination, candidates rotate around stations, allowing between 5 and 20 min at each. In most undergraduate examinations, three to five stations will test clinical examination skills. Other stations may be used for testing factual knowledge, interpretation of growth or laboratory data, and recognition and understanding of clinical photographs and radiology. Most will include a communications station. Here, an actor or member of staff will play the role of a parent. The candidate is expected to discuss a diagnosis or illness with the parent, offering the essential facts in a way that is easy to understand, while demonstrating appropriate empathy and good interpersonal skills.

OSCE stations are given at the end of the chapters. Each one gives the elements that the examiners will expect, common examples and specific notes on that system. In these OSCE stations, we outline clinical examination, assessment of growth, nutrition and physical development, and give details of system examinations.

OSCE station format

Clinical approach:

Here you will find:
- what to check
- how to approach the child
- what to examine
- what to ask
- how to communicate
- technique

In the OSCE, almost all the marks are given for technique. The emphasis is not on making the diagnosis.

The examiner is likely to say:
- complete the examination and tell me what you have found

OR
- as you examine the child, tell me your findings

If not stipulated, you may do either

Here you will find an example of a clinical OSCE station

The question you will be asked
- *please examine.....*
- *please explain.....*
- *please take a history.....*
- *please examine this urine.....*

We give an example of a typical child or clinical problem used in the OSCE.

This box contains the diagnosis in this example, which you may or may not be asked to make

Never forget:

Here you will find:
- HIGHCOST (see below)

Look around for:

Here you will find:
- useful clues
- look at the family, the surroundings
- aids to examination (e.g. toys, rattles)

Special points

Here you will find:
- hints and tips
- how not to upset the child
- special techniques

All OSCE stations begin with HIGHCOST. This acronym emphasizes the importance of the first clinical impression and the findings of simple observation, which are central to good paediatric clinical assessment. Perhaps the acronym will also remind us that good clinical assessment is expensive of time, but highly cost effective!

HIGHCOST

Hello
Introduce yourself
General inspection
Health and hands
Centiles
Obvious
Systems examination
Thank you

Hello

Children are quick to assess adults, and often very accurate. Approach the child with courtesy, a smile and a friendly greeting. There are two essential reasons that every undergraduate should remember this: it is an important clinical skill, and in almost every OSCE examination a student will get marks for it!

Introduce yourself

Introduce yourself and find out to whom you are speaking. What does the child like to be called? Matt may only be called Matthew when his parents are annoyed with him.

General inspection

During the general introduction, and often while taking the clinical history, the doctor will learn a lot about the child, her parents and the relationships between them. You should also note if the child has an unusual appearance or abnormal features which fit into a recognized pattern (e.g. Down's syndrome, achondroplasia).

The doctor should not tower over the child, or lean over them during examination.

The good doctor will note:
• Does the child look well cared for? (Be careful. Some clean, well-behaved children are unloved. Some caring parents choose outrageous clothes and hairstyles for their children.)
• Is there a loving relationship between the child and the parents? Do the parents talk as if the child was not there, or as if she is an inanimate object? Are the parents showing an appropriate level of concern whilst sharing the problem with you?
• Is the child confident or clinging to the parent? Is he crying? When he seeks reassurance from his parent, does he get it? These are difficult assessments, particularly when a child is unwell.
• Does the child have any unusual features? Are the body proportions appropriate? Look at the child's face. Before you commit yourself to a dysmorphic syndrome, look at the parents' faces.

Health and hands
• Is the child ill or well?
• In the young child this is often the most important clinical sign. In the acutely unwell, 6-month-old infant, a pale, listless unresponsive appearance with glazed eyes, has essential implications for diagnosis and immediate management. The experienced parent who simply reports that their child is ill should be listened to carefully. The hospital doctor who receives a phone call from a GP stating that the diagnosis is not clear, but that the child looks ill, should appreciate the urgency and importance of this statement.
• Facial appearance may be helpful. Look

for swelling, pallor, jaundice or cyanosis. Examine the conjunctiva for signs of anaemia.
• Features that raise concern:
   ♦ A child who is inattentive, limp or intermittently distressed.
   ♦ Pallor, mottled skin or the infant who appears grey.
   ♦ Hypoxia may make a child sleepy or agitated. Cyanosis may be hard to see.
   ♦ Dehydration should be assessed (p. 160).
   ♦ Increased work of breathing (p. 141).
   ♦ Fever.
• It is often helpful to start the examination by holding the child's hand. It is not only a friendly gesture, but is often informative.
   ♦ Everyone looks for clubbing. It usually isn't there.
   ♦ Quickly assess the pulse. The radial pulse is commonly used, but in infants the brachial may be easier to feel.
   ♦ Assess perfusion. Are the hands well perfused or cold and clammy.
   ♦ Capillary refill is assessed by gently squeezing the nail so that the nail bed becomes pale. Upon release, the nail bed should again become pink within 2 s. Pale hands may indicate anaemia, which is better assessed from the conjunctiva.

Centiles
The only way to assess these features is by reference to normal population data, most commonly by plotting growth on a centile chart (see below). Brief assessment may be made on simple assessment.

Obvious
• Record observations which are immediately apparent. These include the leg in plaster, the central venous line, the nasogastric tube, ankle/foot orthoses (splints) or a pile of inhalers. Injuries should be recorded. It is surprising how such observations may be forgotten if they are not written down.

Systems examination

In paediatrics, each system does not need to be examined in a fixed order. Often examination of the body systems must be opportunistic. If the toddler is undressed and lying peacefully in his mother's arms, one might begin by listening to the heart. Potentially upsetting procedures (inspection of the throat) should sensibly be left for last. Many children prefer not to be undressed completely, although by the end of examination all parts of the body should have been inspected. In undergraduate examination genitalia should not be examined, except in young infants, and rectal examination should never be performed.

During systems examination, ask about the child's family, friends, pets, hobbies or favourite TV programmes. Show him any instruments you are going to use, and explain how they work.

Thank you

Gratitude for the privilege of examining a child is never misplaced. The family will all appreciate praise for a child's good behaviour and cooperation.

> **i** In the OSCE, concentrate on the system examination required, but do not forget HIGHCOST.

Growth and nutrition

The characteristics of children which most clearly distinguish them from adults are growth (increase in size) and development (organ maturation, sexual development and the acquisition of new skills) (Fig. 3.1).

Growth is best estimated by plotting weight and height (length in babies) on appropriate charts. Rates of increase are good indicators of general health and nutri-

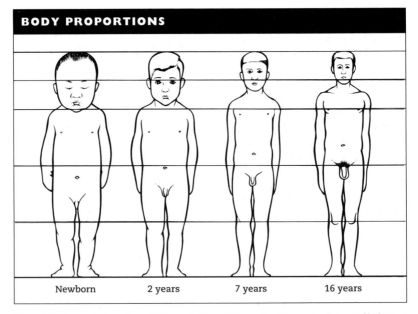

BODY PROPORTIONS

| Newborn | 2 years | 7 years | 16 years |

Fig. 3.1 Body proportions from birth to adulthood. The ratio of the parts above and below the symphysis pubis falls from 1.7 : 1 in the newborn to 0.9 : 1 in the adult.

tion. Children should be weighed either in underclothes (babies in nappies) or naked, but always the same way because changes in weight are more important than absolute values. Height and length are accurately measured with stadiometers which are wall mounted and calibrated. If children are upset at the prospect of being weighed and measured, leave it until the clinical examination is over: tears are more easily prevented than stopped.

Centile charts are constructed from measurements of many children who are free from recognized problems which affect their growth (Fig. 3.2). Modern charts are based on cross-sectional and longitudinal data (Table 3.1; see Fig. 3.3). The difference between an individual's growth and the figures obtained by using measurements from groups of children of different ages is most obvious at puberty. The individual child will first accelerate towards a higher centile, and then gradually level off as the rate of the pubertal growth spurt slows. Full assessment of height may require information about pubertal status and bone age (p. 29). Growth is most rapid in the first year and at puberty, but remarkably constant between.

Accurate nutritional assessment is difficult and complex. The initial clinical impression is usually valuable. An undernourished child is 'all skin and bone'; the limbs are slender, the bony prominences are conspicuous, loss of muscle bulk may be observed. In the younger child this is seen as wasting of the buttocks. Mid-upper arm circumference is measured simply with a tape measure around the arm at the mid point between the elbow and the shoulder. Centile charts provide reference data but, in the child aged 1–5 years, a circumference less than 14 cm suggests poor nutrition and needs further assessment. If weight loss has been recent, folds of skin on the lower abdomen and inner aspects of the thighs may be seen.

Excess fat is most evident on the trunk. Fat can be measured using skinfold thickness, measured with calipers. Weight for height can be assessed by looking at the relative centiles for the two measurements.

> Bodymass index [BMI = weight (kg) ÷ height (m)^2] varies with age and charts are now available. BMI >20 in a child of 1–10 years indicates obesity.

Other useful measurements include sitting height (which reflects body proportions), and arm span (which is usually similar to height).

Dental development

The average ages of eruption of the teeth are shown below but there is a wide normal range.

There are 20 deciduous and 32 permanent teeth; permanent teeth appear from the 6th year. The first molars and central incisors appear first. All teeth have appeared by the age of 14 except the third molars. Teeth appear a few months earlier in girls (Table 3.2).

HEAD CIRCUMFERENCE

Head circumference (cm) centile table

	2%	50%	98%
Birth	33	35	38
12 months	43	47	49
18 months	45	49	51
2 years	46	50	52
3 years	47	50	53
5 years	48	51	54
8 years	50	52	55
12 years	51	54	56
14 years	52	56	58

Table 3.1 Normal head circumference.

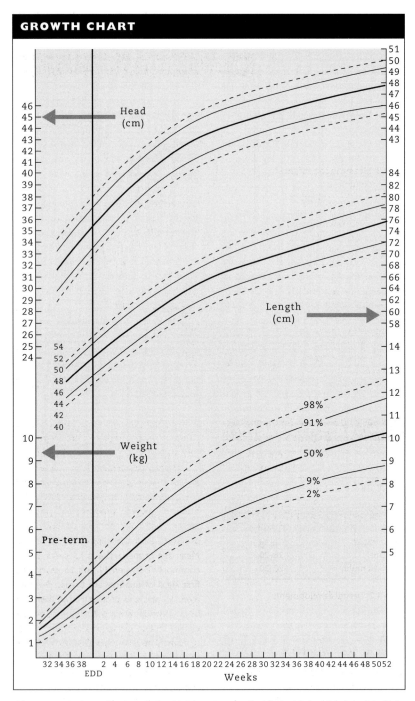

Fig. 3.2 A growth centile chart for head circumference, length (height) and weight. Similar charts are available for various age ranges and each sex.

HEAD MEASUREMENT

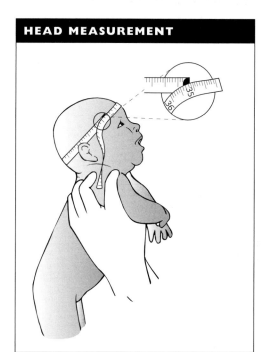

Fig. 3.3 Measuring an infant's head circumference.

- *head circumference* is an important measurement, and reflects the volume of the cranial contents with surprising accuracy;
- a good quality, inelastic tape is used;
- the tape passes over the occiput, above the ears, and the prominence of the brow;
- two or three measurements are taken in slightly different planes, and the largest is recorded as the head circumference.

DENTAL DEVELOPMENT

Deciduous		Appearance (months)
Central incisor	Lower	6–10
	Upper	7–10
Lateral incisor	Upper	8–10
	Lower	12–18
First molar		12–18
Canine		16–20
Second molar		20–30

Table 3.2 Dental development.

Sexual development

Human sexual development is concentrated into two brief periods of time: Primary sexual development in the embryo and the appearance of secondary sex characteristics during puberty (Fig 3.4).

At puberty, changes occur in response to pituitary gonadotrophins. The trigger for release of these hormones is still unknown. The age of onset of puberty is very variable and is influenced by racial, hereditary and nutritional factors. In girls in the UK today, breast development begins at 11 years on average, and pubic hair a little later. Early breast development may be asymmetrical. Mean age of menarche is 13 years, but is commonly between 11 and 15 years. The first signs of puberty are breast development in girls and growth of the testes in boys. In both sexes, puberty is accompanied by an impressive growth spurt, which is maximal in girls at age 12 years, and boys at 14 years. The progress of puberty is recorded in stages of pubic hair (both sexes), external genitalia (male) and breast development (female) (Figs 3.5 and 3.6). Epiphyseal fusion, with cessation of growth, marks the end of puberty.

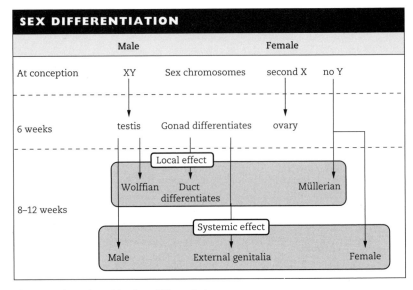

Fig. 3.4 Embryonic and fetal sex differentiation.

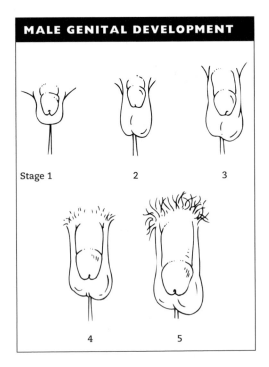

Fig. 3.5 Stages of male genital development.
(1) Preadolescent.
(2) Enlargement of scrotum and testes.
(3) Increases of breadth of penis and development of glans.
(4) Testes continue to enlarge. Scrotum darkens.
(5) Adult: by this time pubic hair has spread to medial surface of thighs.

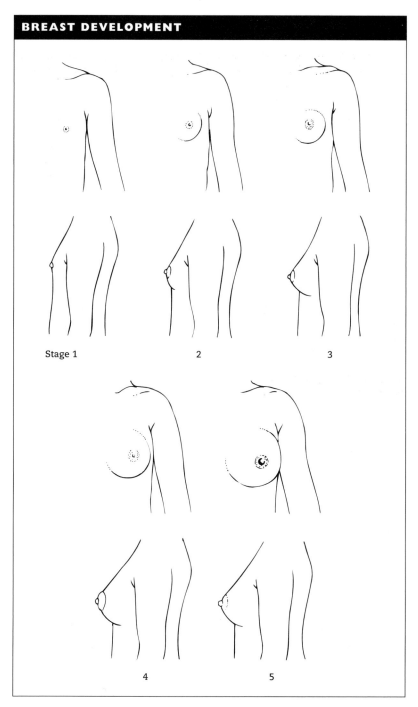

Fig. 3.6 Stages of breast development. (1) Pre-adolescent—elevation of papilla only. (2) Breast bud stage. (3) Further enlargement of breast and areola. (4) Projection of areola and papilla above level of breast. (5) Mature stage—areola has recessed, papilla projects.

Bone age (or skeletal age) is a useful index of growth and maturation. A plain X-ray of the hand and wrist is taken. Calcification of the epiphyses, and later their fusion, is noted for each of the bones around the wrist, and compared with standard pictures. The method is complex and requires special skills. In healthy children bone age relates more closely to height than to age, short children tending to have 'delayed', and tall children 'advanced' bone ages. Significant advance or delay in bone age merits investigation.

Systems examination

Head and neck

- Superficial lymph glands are always palpable in the neck and groins of children. Normal glands are soft, mobile, non-tender and usually not larger than an acorn. Enlarged tonsillar glands, just behind the angle of the jaw, indicate past or present throat infections. Generalized lymphadenopathy suggests systemic illness unless it is due to widespread skin disease (e.g. eczema).

Changes in the fontanelle may be important clues if supported by other clinical signs:

Large fontanelle → hydrocephalus
Small fontanelle → slow brain growth
Sunken fontanelle → dehydration
Bulging fontanelle → raised intracranial pressure

- Jaundice may be difficult to detect, especially in artificial lighting.
- The *anterior fontanelle* is widely open at birth, but varies considerably in size. It closes between 9 and 18 months.
    - Gentle pressure over the fontanelle gives an indication of its tension. The normal fontanelle is relaxed when the infant is resting. It pulsates with the heartbeat. Tension increases when the infant cries or strains.
- The *posterior fontanelle* is far back where the sagittal and lambdoid sutures meet. It closes soon after birth.
- A *third fontanelle* is sometimes present in the sagittal suture just in front of the posterior fontanelle. It may be a marker for other congenital abnormality.

Ear, nose and throat

This is an important part of the general examination of any child, especially an ill child. It is difficult in babies, and young children may dislike having their ears examined. Practice makes perfect. The infant will be happier if securely held and this prevents accidental damage to the meatus with the speculum (Fig. 3.7).
- The pinna is drawn gently upwards and backwards to allow a clear view of the eardrums.
- If it is essential to view the drum, wax obscuring the view may be removed with a wax hook or a cotton wool bud. This procedure should not be attempted unless the child is quiet and the doctor skilled.
- The nasal mucosa may be examined with the auroscope. Note the colour of the mucosa, the presence of oedema and secretions.
- Examine the mouth, noting the state of the gums, teeth, tongue and buccal mucosa.
- If children will put their tongue out and say 'ah', posterior pharynx may be viewed without a tongue depressor. A wooden tongue depressor is well tolerated by most children. It must be used gently, and not placed so far back as to cause gagging. It is difficult to get a good view of the throat in babies.
- Never use force to view the throat of a young child with stridor: it may precipitate respiratory obstruction.

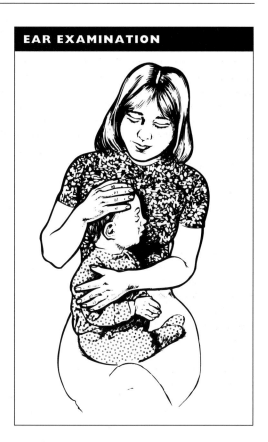

EAR EXAMINATION

Fig. 3.7 Examination of the ear is easier and safer if the infant is held correctly.

Chest and lungs

Inspect the chest

• *Hyperinflation* is caused by chronic obstructive airways disease as in bad asthma, or seen acutely in conditions like bronchiolitis.

• *Pectus carinatum*: the sternum is displaced forward, relative to the ribs. Children do not like to hear themselves referred to as pigeon-chested.

• *Pectus excavatum*: a depression in the anterior chest wall above the epigastrium due to a short central tendon of the diaphragm which tethers the lower end of the sternum.

• *Harrison's sulcus*. Indrawing of the lower rib caused by the diaphragm in conditions such as severe asthma. This is a linear indentation, parallel and just above the costal margin.

Assess respiratory effort

• Respiratory rate. Tachypnoea is important. Breathing should be measured at rest over a full 30 s. Normal respiratory rate falls with age: in infants it should be less than 60 per minute, in children it should be less than 40 per minute.

• Rates less than 20 or intermittent apnoea should always raise immediate and urgent concern.

• Pattern of breathing. Prolonged expiration occurs with wheeze. Deep, sighing (acidotic) breathing occurs in diabetic ketoacidosis and salicylate poisoning.
• Recession in the intercostal spaces, epigastrium and suprasternal notch may be seen with increased respiratory effort and obstruction of airflow into the lungs.
• Nasal flaring.
• Grunting on expiration.
• Difficulties in walking, talking, drinking or speaking.

Detect added noises
• Wheeze: a predominantly expiratory sound, due to obstruction in the lower airways. Typical of asthma and bronchiolitis.
• Stridor: a predominantly inspiratory sound, indicating upper airway obstruction and typical of croup or laryngeal oedema.
• Cough: most often arises in the upper respiratory tract. Children tend to swallow sputum rather than spit it out. A barking cough is typical of croup. Paroxysms of coughing occur in whooping cough.

Percussion
Place finger firmly, but gently, in contact with the anterior chest wall. Percuss your own finger lightly. Percuss over the clavicle and the front of the chest and in three positions on each side of the chest posteriorly.

Auscultation
Use an appropriate sized stethoscope. An adult-sized stethoscope placed on a newborn baby will pick up heart, breath and bowel sounds all at once! Compare air entry on both sides. In small children, it is normal for breath sounds to be bronchial.
• If a young child finds it hard to take a deep breath, ask them to blow out, and listen when they breathe in afterwards.
• Coarse crepitations are often transmitted from the throat or upper airways. These may clear if the child coughs first.

Cardiovascular system

Inspection
• Look for increased respiratory rate or other signs of increased work of breathing.
• Watch a baby feeding. Poor feeding is a cardinal sign of heart failure. The infant sucks well at first, but then has to stop for a rest.
• Is there cyanosis on rest or on exertion?
• Precordial bulge: the right ventricle pushes the sternum forward.
• Ventricular heave: the right ventricle causes the lower sternum to move forward with each cardiac impulse.

Pulse
• The minimum requirement is to count the pulse and to examine its character in both brachials. Check that the femoral pulses are present and that there is no brachio-femoral delay.
• Young infants show sinus dysrhythmia: heart rate increases in inspiration.
• Rate
• Rhythm
• Character. Small volume in shock; bounding pulse in patent ductus arteriosis.

Palpation
• Find the apex beat. It should be in the 4th or 5th intercostal space, just lateral to the nipple.
• Check the apex is on the left.
• Thrills are the vibration of a loud murmur. If you do not hear a murmur, you have not felt a thrill.

Auscultation
• Listen for two heart sounds.
• Splitting of the second sound is easily heard in children and is usually normal. The gap between the aortic and pulmonary second sounds increases in inspiration.
• A third heart sound is often heard at the cardiac apex.

Murmurs

- Timing: pansystolic, ejection systolic, continuous or, rarely, diastolic.
- Quality: describe the sound or character.
- Site of maximum intensity: where?
- Intensity: how loud is it?
- Radiation: can the murmur be heard in the neck or back?

INTENSITY GRADING OF HEART MURMUR

1 Barely audible
2 Soft
3 Easy to hear, no thrill
4 Loud, easily audible, thrill
5 Very loud, with easily palpable thrill
6 Audible with the stethoscope held off the chest

Blood pressure

The cuff should be wide enough to cover two thirds of the distance between the tip of the elbow and shoulder. Too small a cuff yields a falsely high blood pressure. Blood pressure may be determined by auscultation.

Automated methods (e.g. Dinamap) using the oscillometeric principle are commonly used in paediatrics.

In the neonatal period mean systolic blood pressure is 70 mm Hg. From 6 weeks to 10 years of age, mean systolic blood pressure remains around 95 mm Hg, and most children will have a systolic blood pressure less than 115 mm Hg. Mean systolic blood pressure is 125 mm Hg by 16 years of age.

Abdomen and gastrointestinal tract

Mouth

- The oral cavity should be examined thoroughly. Note cracking and soreness around the lips.

Inspection

- Abdominal distention
- Normal toddlers are rather pot bellied. The mother will be able to say whether the abdomen is swollen.
- Visible peristalsis
- Hernia
- The acutely painful abdomen does not move normally with respiration.

Palpation

- Is the abdomen soft or tender with guarding? Palpate gently and then more deeply whilst talking to the child and carefully observing for signs of tenderness in the abdomen and on the child's face.
- **Hernia.** Umbilical hernia is easily seen. Inguinal hernias may not be immediately evident; femoral hernias are hard to find.
- **Hepatomegaly.** The liver is normally palpable 1–2 cm below the costal margin in infants and young children.
    ♦ Palpate from the left iliac fossa upwards. The liver edge moves down with the respiration.
    ♦ Percussion may be helpful.
    ♦ Size of the liver is measured below the costal margin in the mid-clavicular line.
- **Splenomegaly.** The spleen tip may be felt in young infants. Palpate from the right iliac fossa, across the abdomen.
    ♦ Spleen moves downwards or diagonally on respiration. The notch is palpable. One cannot get above it, and it is felt anteriorly.
- **Renal swelling**
    ♦ Normal kidneys may be palpable in the newborn period.
    ♦ Kidneys felt bimanually.
    ♦ Kidneys move down with respiration.

Ascites

- Diffuse swelling
- Shifting dullness: gas filled bowel produces resonant percussion note on the uppermost point of the abdomen.
- If ascites is present: when the child lies on

his back, the abdomen is resonant around the umbilicus and dull in the flanks. Turn the child so that one side is uppermost. The upper flank should now be resonant and the umbilical area dull (Fig. 3.8).
• Faecal masses are frequently felt in the line of the colon and in the left iliac fossa.

Percussion
• The liver and large spleen are dull to percussion. Shifting dullness demonstrates ascites.

Auscultation
• Increased bowel sounds: intestinal hurry, e.g. gastroenteritis and early intestinal obstruction.
• Decreased bowel sounds: paralytic ileus.

Rectal examination
Rectal examination is rarely indicated in children. It should only be performed by a skilled doctor who can interpret the findings.

Examine stool for colour, consistency and the presence of blood or mucus.

Urinalysis
• Urine should be examined and tested with a multireagent stick (p. 200).

Genitalia

Boys
• Is the penis a normal shape? Is the urethral meatus at the tip of the penis or displaced (hypospadias, epispadias).
• Scrotum and testes. The retractile testis is drawn back up into the scrotum in response to cutaneous stimulation: this is normal in small boys. Determine if testes are undescended or ectopic.
• Scrotal swelling may be fluid (hydrocele) or hernia.

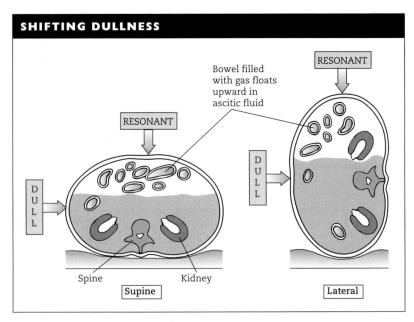

SHIFTING DULLNESS

Bowel filled with gas floats upward in ascitic fluid

RESONANT

RESONANT

DULL

DULL

Spine   Kidney

Supine

Lateral

Fig. 3.8 Schematic diagram of shifting dullness. Dullness to percussion shifts as the fluid moves and the bowel floats.

Girls
• Examine vulva and external genitalia.
• Look for soreness, injury, discharge, or abnormalities.

Neurology

"All that is needed is space and time: space for the child to run around and time to watch him." (Dr Stuart Green)

Motor function

Activity
• Formal examination of tone, power and coordination should be used to help confirm or explain the findings made on simple observation (Table 3.3).
• Does the infant show appropriate head control for age? Is the small child floppy when picked up? Is there symmetry and normal patterns of movement? Can the older child walk or run? Ask the child to sit on the floor and rise quickly. Can the child walk on tip toe or on his heels?
• These observations should be made before reaching for the tendon hammer. Check with the mother first, and encourage a child gently. If a child is unable to walk, asking him to do so is not kind.

Muscle tone
• The normal infant and young child can touch his ears with his toes. Observe head control and look for hypotonia when the infant is picked up.
• Muscle tone is generally assessed on passive movement. Ensure the child is relaxed.
• The commonest abnormality of tone is *spasticity* (increased tone around a joint in one direction of movement). The commonest groups of muscles affected are the hip adductors (test by abducting the hips) and the plantar flexors (tested by dorsi-flexing the foot). When both groups are affected, scissoring and toe pointing is seen.

Muscle power
This is best tested in children old enough to cooperate by giving simple commands, e.g. 'squeeze my fingers', 'push me away'. Formal grading of muscle power is seldom used in young children. It is best to describe effects of abnormal power on movement and activity.

Muscle wasting
Loss of muscle bulk may be seen in a wide variety of disorders. Hypertrophy of the calf muscles is seen in Duchenne muscular dystrophy (Fig. 3.9).

Tendon reflexes and clonus
Reflexes are often easier to elicit in a child than an adult. The child must be relaxed. Reinforcement may be helpful: ask the child to squeeze his hands together.

Table 3.3 Characteristics of upper and lower motor neurone lesions.

MOTOR NEURONE LESIONS

	Upper motor neurone	Lower motor neurone
Example	Cerebral palsy	Spina bifida
Strength	Decreased	Decreased
Tone	Increased	Decreased
Reflexes	Increased	Absent/decreased
Clonus	Present	Absent

GOWER'S SIGN

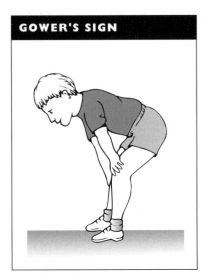

Fig. 3.9 Gower's sign. If asked to rise from sitting on the floor, the child turns prone and climbs up his own legs. This indicates limb girdle weakness and is typical of Duchenne dystrophy.

Brisk reflexes in association with spasticity suggest an upper motor neurone (pyramidal) lesion.

Plantar response may be extensor in the normal child until around the age of walking. In older children, a normal flexor response should be seen.

Ankle clonus, if sustained, is suggestive of an upper motor neurone lesion. It is best tested for with the knee semiflexed. Dorsiflex the ankle sharply, trying different degrees of pressure. Pressing too lightly or too hard may mask clonus.

Coordination

This may be tested in children more than 2 years old by the finger–nose and heel–shin manoeuvres. In younger children it is more helpful to watch for any unsteadiness when playing. A healthy 3-year-old can stand on one leg briefly, and make a good attempt to walk heel-to-toe along a straight line on the floor.

To test for *dysdiadochokinesis*, ask the child to copy you patting the back of one hand as fast as possible, and then the other. Even 10 year olds cannot do it as fast as an adult can.

Sensation and proprioception

A child who has significant abnormalities in this area is likely to show problems when observed in general activities. Full testing of sensation is rarely performed. It is very difficult in infants and toddlers, but enjoyed by older children. Painful stimuli should not be used.

Cranial nerves

Examination often includes inspection of the eyes, external ocular movement and observation for manifest squint (p. 102).

Facial nerve function and hearing should be observed. Other tests are only performed if there is indication (Table 3.4).

Ophthalmoscopy and examination of the fundi is difficult. Looking at the optic disk has been described as 'trying to identify a friend on a passing Intercity train'. Ask the child to fix on an object in a dimly lit room, and make sure the ophthalmoscope light is not too bright. With patience, the disk can often be seen. Do not worry if you fail — you are in good company!

The eye should also be inspected for corneal opacity, abnormality or cataract. If good visualization of the retina is essential in young children, consider referral to the ophthalmologist.

Examination of bones and joints

Fractures and bone infections are common in childhood and will cause local pain, tenderness and sometimes swelling. Joint disease is not so common, but arthritis

NERVE FUNCTION TESTS

Nerve	Function	Test
I	Smell	Not often tested
II	Acuity	Simple tests of vision appropriate for age
	Pupils	Direct and consensual light reflex
	Fields	Facing child, who is fixing on your face, test peripheral vision horizontally and vertically
	Squint	See p. 99
III IV VI }	External ocular movements	Facing child, watch following of bright object in H pattern. In infants and toddlers, head may be held
V	Masseter	Clench jaw
	Sensation	Light touch on face (avoid corneal reflex)
VII	Facial muscles	Observe smiling or crying. Ask child to show teeth, close eyes tight, and watch eyebrows during upward gaze
VIII	Hearing	8 months: distraction testing. Pre-school: cooperation testing. Over 5 years: audiometry. All ages: tympanometry, auditory evoked responses. Ask parents: is she deaf?
IX X }	Swallowing, palate, larynx	Observe swallowing, listen to voice, inspect palatal movement
XI	Trapezius	Ask child to shrug
XII	Tongue	Ask child to stick out tongue and move it from side to side

Table 3.4 Tests for nerve function.

and synovitis do occur. Each joint must be examined carefully:

• *Inspection*: is there swelling or deformity? Does the skin look red? Compare the two sides. Is there wasting of adjacent muscles? If in doubt, measure. If a joint is painful, ask the child to show you how far it will move without pain before you touch it.

• *Palpation*: does the skin feel hot? Is there tenderness? Is there fluid in the joint? Is there crepitus when the joint moves? Put the joint through the full range of movement in every direction, watching the child's face to be sure you do not hurt him. Compare the two sides.

• *Measurement*: comparison of muscle bulk can be made by measuring the greatest circumference of the calves, upper arm or forearm muscles. Thighs should be measured about their middle, marking the same distance above the patella on the two sides. Leg lengths are measured with the legs in line with the trunk, from the anterior superior iliac spine or the umbilicus to the medial malleolus at the ankle, taking the tape medial to the patella.

Joint movements

Joint movement should be tested gently if pain may be present. Active and passive range of movement should be noted. The *hip* movements are internal and external rotation, adduction, abduction, flexion and extension. Hip disease may be associated with buttock wasting and/or leg shortening. All newborns are tested for congenital dislocation of the hip (p. 179).

The *knee* normally extends beyond 180° and flexes until the heel touches the buttock. Knee disease is often associated with quadriceps wasting.

The *spine* should be examined for abnormal curvature and for mobility.

OSCE Station: Counselling

Clinical approach:

- read any facts given to you
- have mental/written list of main points
- ask open questions at beginning and end (e.g. is there anything else you would like me to talk about?)
- note reasons for special concern (e.g. other member of family with same problem)
- deal with common concerns
- remember body language—yours and the mother's
- listen
- it may help to write down the diagnosis, or draw a diagram

Information to give

- diagnosis, description of problem
- what do we know
- the cause
- explain the child's symptoms
- what can be done
- how will it affect the child
- what treatment
- what investigations
- follow up

Please talk to this mother. Her 3-year-old son had a febrile convulsion 2 days ago and is now well. She would like to discuss this with you before going home

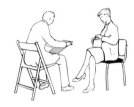

- listen to what she knows
- explain diagnosis
  - ◇ fit caused by fever in healthy child
  - ◇ 6 months—5 years of age
- common (3% of all children)
- fits are frightening but seldom dangerous
  - ◇ how did parents feel during child's fit?
  - ◇ many parents think that their child is dying
- prognosis good
  - ◇ most have no more febrile fits
  - ◇ one third will have a second episode
  - ◇ epilepsy rare
- prevention
  - ◇ recognition of fever
  - ◇ light clothing, antipyretic, tepid sponging
- further fits
  - ◇ first aid
  - ◇ when to seek help

Member of staff is likely to play role of mother
The child is not present

Never forget:

- say hello and introduce yourself
- general health— is the child ill?
- empathic enquiry: how is Sally today?
- are you and the child's parent comfortable?

Look around for:

- hospital records
- information leaflets

Special points

- in some exams, you will be given a history first
- listen for hints to unexpressed worries
- 'parent' is probably a hospital secretary —you usually do not need to put your arm round them

Developmental Assessment

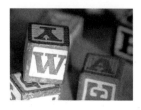

Healthy development has a wide range of 'normal'. The main purposes of developmental assessment are:

• early detection of significant delay so that help (advice, physiotherapy, spectacles, hearing aid) can be provided early

• to provide reassurance to parents.

There are two parts to a developmental assessment, the history presented by the mother and the doctor's own observations. The history is usually reliable and augments the clinical examination, but parents may exaggerate their child's abilities or misinterpret involuntary movements.

I *The history.* The mother should be encouraged to give a careful account of the child's *present skills*, ensuring that each of the four main categories is covered. If there are older siblings, it is helpful to enquire how the child's skills compare with those of the siblings at that age. Enquire about school performance if the child is at school for she is unlikely to have a significant developmental problem if she is coping well in a normal class of children of similar age. *Past history*—Try to obtain information about the dates of the early milestones. Some mothers recall them well, others not at all. If an experienced mother says 'she was very quick', it may not be necessary to obtain exact detail of past achievements.

2 *Play with the child*—in the presence of the parent so as to encourage the child to show certain skills.

Try to define the limit of achievement by noting both the skills the child has and those he has not. The following simple tests require equipment that is available in any surgery or clinic, and require no special expertise on the part of the examiner. They are screening tests which indentify children who need more detailed expert assessment. The ages given are the *average* ages at which the skill is seen.

FOUR AREAS OF DEVELOPMENT

• Posture and movement
• Vision and manipulation
• Hearing and speech
• Social and play

The first 4 months

This is the most difficult time to assess the baby, because it is not until about 6 months that many of the easier developmental tests can be used. Therefore, developmental testing before the age of 6 months is less reliable than at any other time.

Posture and movement (gross motor)

Body control is acquired from the top downwards:

• *Head on trunk*—the newborn baby held upright can balance his head briefly. Laid on his back and pulled up by arms or shoulders, there is complete head lag. By 4 months the head comes up in line with the trunk. By 6 months the head comes up in advance of the trunk.

• *Trunk on pelvis*—by 7 months a baby can sit briefly on a firm, flat surface, often using his arms for support. By 9 months he sits without arm support and can turn without falling.

• *Pelvis on legs*—by 10 months he can pull himself up to stand and begins to cruise round the furniture. By 12–15 months he can walk unaided.

Vision and manipulation (fine motor/adaptive)

Visual attention

At 8 weeks a baby observes with a convergent gaze a dangling toy or bright object held 20–30 cm (9–12 inches) from his face, and moves his head and neck in order to follow it. A true squint (as distinct from a pseudo-squint as seen with epicanthic folds) is always abnormal and requires referral to a specialist (p. 99).

From 2 months a baby prefers to watch a face rather than anything else. The ability to fix and follow improves and can be tested by watching the baby follow a rolling ball, the toddler matching toys, or the 5-year-old matching letters.

Grasp

A wooden tongue depressor is held before the infant. At 6 months he approaches it with the ulnar border of the hand and then takes it in a clumsy *palmar grasp*. At 9 months he approaches it with the radial border and takes it in a *scissor grasp* between the sides of thumb and index finger before transferring it to the other hand and putting in his mouth. At 12 months he approaches it with the index finger and picks it up precisely between the ends of the thumb and index finger in a *pincer grasp*. Once the pincer grasp is developed, parents notice that their child can pick up the tiniest bits of fluff on the carpet (Fig. 4.1).

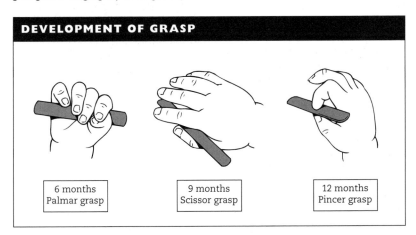

DEVELOPMENT OF GRASP

| 6 months Palmar grasp | 9 months Scissor grasp | 12 months Pincer grasp |

Fig. 4.1 Development of grasp.

Copying

A child will copy with a pencil the following shapes:

l or — at 2 years	□ at 5 years
O at 3 years	△ at 6 years
+ at 4 years	◊ at 7 years

Hearing and speech (language)

Localization of sounds (distraction test)

The baby is sat on mother's knee facing another adult about 3 m (10 feet) away whose function is to keep the baby's visual

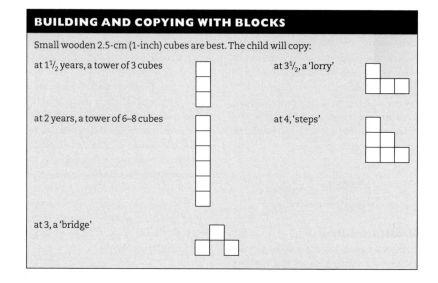

BUILDING AND COPYING WITH BLOCKS

Small wooden 2.5-cm (1-inch) cubes are best. The child will copy:

at 1½ years, a tower of 3 cubes

at 2 years, a tower of 6–8 cubes

at 3, a 'bridge'

at 3½, a 'lorry'

at 4, 'steps'

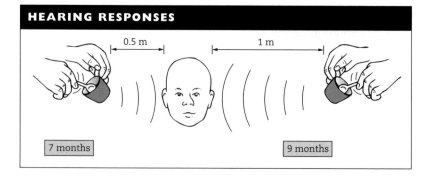

HEARING RESPONSES

0.5 m

1 m

7 months

9 months

Fig. 4.2 Hearing responses in the first year. At 7 months, the sound should be made 0.5 m lateral to the ear. From 9 months, the sound should be made 1 m lateral to the ear.

DEVELOPMENTAL MILESTONES

Posture and movement	Vision and manipulation
3 months	
Prone: rests on forearms lifts up head and chest	Vision: alert, watches movement of adult
Pulled to sit: head bobs forwards, then held erect	Follows dangling toy held 15 cm from face
Held standing sags at knees	Hands: loosely open
6 months	
Sits erect with support	Reaches out for toy and takes in palmar grasp, puts to mouth
Prone: lifts up on extended arms	Transfers object from hand to hand
Held standing: takes weight on legs	Watches rolling ball 2 m away
9 months	
Sits unsupported for 10 minutes	Scissor grasp
Prone: wriggles or crawls	Looks for toys that are dropped
Held standing: bounces or stamps	
12 months	
Walks round furniture stepping sideways (cruising)	Index finger approach to tiny objects then pincer grasp
Crawls on all fours; walks with hands held	Drops toys deliberately and watches where they go
18 months	
Walks alone and can pick up a toy from floor without falling	Builds tower of three cubes
	Scribbles
2 years	
Runs	Builds tower of six cubes
Walks up and down stairs two feet to a step	
3 years	
Walks upstairs one foot per step, and down two feet per step	Builds tower of nine cubes
Stands on one foot momentarily	Copies an O
4 years	
Walks up and down stairs one foot per step	Builds three steps from six cubes (after demonstration)
Stands on one foot for 5 s	Copies O and X
5 years	
Skips, hops	Draws a man
Stands on one foot with arms folded for 5 seconds	Copies O, X and □

Table 4.1 Developmental milestones (average age of achievements). *Continued on p. 46.*

DEVELOPMENTAL MILESTONES

Hearing and speech	Social behaviour
3 months Chuckles and coos when pleased Quietens to interesting sounds	Shows pleasure appropriately
6 months Makes double syllable sounds and tuneful noises (gurgles) Localizes soft sounds 45 cm (15 inches) lateral to either ear	Alert, interested Still friendly with strangers
9 months Babbles tunefully Brisk localization of soft sounds 1 m (3 feet) lateral to either ear	Distinguishes strangers and shows apprehension Chews solids
12 months Babbles incessantly A few words Understands simple commands	Cooperates with dressing, e.g. holding up arms Waves bye bye
18 months Uses many words, sound labels Occasionally two words together	Drinks from cup using two hands Demands constant mothering
2 years Joins words together in simple phrases, as sound ideas	Uses spoon Indicates toilet needs, dry by day Play imitates adult activities
3 years Speaks in sentences Gives full name	Eats with spoon and fork Can undress with assistance Dry by night
4 years Talks a lot Speech contains many infantile substitutions	Dresses and undresses with assistance
5 years Fluent speech with few infantile substitutions	Dresses and undresses alone Washes and dries face and hands

attention straight ahead (but without being so fascinating that the baby ignores the test sounds).

A variety of soft sounds are made lateral to either ear and out of the line of vision. Rustling tissue provides a high-frequency sound; a spoon gently scraped round a cup, or a high-pitched rattle are other suitable sounds. Provided the baby has reasonable hearing she will turn to locate the source. At 7 months the baby turns to sounds 0.5 m from either ear. At 9 months he turns promptly to sounds 1 m away. The optimal age at which to test an infant's hearing is 7 months (Fig. 4.2).

Speech

At 3 months open vowel sounds (ooh, eeh) are made, and consonants by 6 months (goo, gah) — gurgling. By 9 months there is varied and tuneful babbling. From 1 year single word labels are used for familiar objects and people — 'Mum', 'Dog'. At 2 years words are joined to convey ideas — 'Dadad gone' and the child will follow simple instructions, e.g. 'Put the spoon in the cup'. At 3, sentences are used to describe present and past happenings. Throughout this period the child's understanding of language is far ahead of his ability to utter it.

Social behaviour (personal—social)

Smiling

Seen at 4–8 weeks in response to mother's face.

Reacting to strangers

Up to 9 months most babies will be handled happily by anyone; from 9 months they begin to cry or fret if handled by a stranger.

Feeding

At 9 months, lumpy food is chewed. At 18 months, the child cooperates with feeding, and drinks from an ordinary cup using two hands. At 3 years, he can feed himself efficiently with a spoon and fork (Table 4.1).

Limitations of developmental assessment

Technique

As with any examination the expert will get the most reliable information, but anyone who is willing to listen to the mother and observe the child can get some useful information about each of the four main fields of development. If the mother's account differs greatly from what is observed, it may be that the child is having an 'off day', in which case observing on another occasion will be more reliable.

Range of normal

The age at which a normal child achieves a particular physical or developmental goal is extremely variable; 50% of children can walk 10 steps unaided at 13 months, but a few can do this at 8 months, and others not until 18 months. It is kinder to talk to parents of the 'usual' age for developing a skill rather than the 'normal', since abnormal implies a fault, quite commonly one field of activity appears delayed in a normal child, but it is rare for all four fields of development to be delayed if the child is normal. In the preterm infant, correct age for gestation before assessing development.

Milestones are stepping stones

Parents tend to think of certain developmental skills as essential milestones. It is truer to regard them as stepping stones. In general one cannot reach a particular stepping stone without using the previous ones — and a child does not run until she can walk or walk until she can stand. But different people may use different stepping stones, and occasionally miss one out. Most children crawl before they stand, but some shuffle on their bottoms, never crawl, yet stand and walk normally in the end. *Bottom shuffling* is a typical example of the sort of variation in development that can cause parents unnecessary worry, particularly as bottom shufflers tend to walk later than other children.

Using stepping stones we may go in sudden bounds rather than at an even rate—children often develop that way, appearing static for a few weeks then suddenly mastering a new skill. If the next stepping stone is a particularly hard one, all the child's energy may appear to be devoted to just one of the four areas of development, whilst the other three seem static; posture and movement skills may advance rapidly about the age of 1 year as walking is mastered, whilst hearing and speech development appear static.

Whether we like it or not, many parents view their child's developmental assessment in the same way as an undergraduate examination, and all parents want their child to 'pass'. Therefore:

- when we 'test' beyond expected skills—reassure that we do not expect the 9–12-month-old child to walk
- announce 'results' early—if development is normal, say so
- handle 'failure' carefully—be sure before you diagnose delay
- remember that all 'candidates' can have an off day—interpretation is difficult during illness.

OSCE Station: Developmental assessment

Clinical approach:

- combine history, observation and clinical testing
  ◦ watch the child playing
  ◦ think of four areas of development
- assessment of four areas:
  ◦ **gross motor/posture and movement**
  ◦ **fine motor/vision and manipulation**
  ◦ **hearing and speech**
  ◦ **social**
- think in 3–month intervals
- in each area of development:
  ◦ find a skill that the child can do
  ◦ find a more advanced skill that the child cannot do
  ◦ developmental age is between the two
- use any set of recognized milestones
- present findings for each area of development
- summarize your findings

This is Rachel and her mother. Please perform a developmental assessment and tell me how old she is

Posture and Movement

sits supported
rolls over
not cruising
not walking

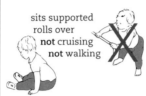

Vision and Manipulation

index approach
scissor grip
transfers
not pincer grip

Hearing and Speech

passed health visitor test
turns to sound
babbles—
lots of sounds
NO words

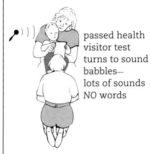

Social

waves bye
holds, bites, chews biscuit
holds bottle when feeding
NOT handing things back
STILL mouthing

Rachel is a healthy child of 10 months

Never forget:

- say hello and introduce yourself
- general health—is the child ill?
- quickly assess growth, nutrition, and development
- mention the obvious (e.g. bandage on arm)

Look around for:

- walking aids
- hearing aids evidence of feeding problems
- glasses
- adapted buggy

Special points

- praise the things a child can do and reassure them when they cannot perform
- developmental age may not be the same in each of the four areas—this can be normal
- did the child perform to her ability?
- children in the developmental OSCE are usually normal healthy children
- as soon as development is considered, start observing the child—they may perform brilliantly until you begin formal assessment, and then go on strike!

Fetal Medicine

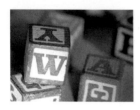

Traditionally, paediatricians have been concerned with children from the moment of their birth, while obstetricians have expressed their concern for the fetus indirectly through their care of the mother. This approach has been quietly revolutionized since the 1960s when thalidomide, a drug taken to relieve vomiting in pregnancy, led to severe fetal limb abnormalities. Fetal medicine was born: primarily an obstetric specialty, but one which demands good collaboration with paediatrics. The expectations of the couple wishing to have a baby have increased in parallel with the advances in fetal medicine and the newer techniques available: ultrasound, amniocentesis, chorionic villus sampling, fetal blood sampling, DNA analysis, fetoscopy and fetal intervention. Risk of Down's syndrome, for example, is assessed using a range of tests including karyotyping, ultrasound, and the triple test (levels of alphafetoprotein, gonadotrophin and oestriol in maternal blood). This has brought with it new diagnostic, management and ethical problems.

Contraception

It is important to appreciate the relationship between contraception and child health. This may sound paradoxical, but high birth rates and high child mortality tend to go hand in hand. In developing countries, large families are usual in the hope that a few will survive to adult life. Medical care reduces mortality from disease, but unless family size is reduced *pari passu*, the children may die from starvation instead. The theory is simple: its translation into practice depends upon the availability of safe, effective, cheap contraception coupled with education of the community to accept it. In Europe, the challenge of providing good, supportive advice to teenagers is widely acknowledged.

Infertility treatment

Methods of helping infertile couples continue to advance. Techniques of ovulation control, *in vitro* fertilization, prolonged storage of gametes and the embryo, and surrogacy permit the separation of functions previously regarded as inseparable:
- production of ova
- sperm production
- place of fertilization
- the uterus in which the fetus develops
- the adult(s) responsible for rearing the child.

Hence the ovum could come from Ms A, be fertilized in the laboratory by sperm from

Mr B, be implanted in the uterus of Ms C and be reared by Mr and Ms D. Doctors need to be aware of the likely effects on the child of the more bizarre variations on this theme. Infertility treatment leads to increased numbers of multiple pregnancies. These infants deliver preterm, with important implications for the infants and the health service.

Antenatal and pre-pregnancy care

Preparation for a baby requires the good physical and emotional health of both parents. Hereditary conditions should be discussed. Women should be immunized against rubella before conception. All but the most essential drugs should be stopped before pregnancy. Smoking and alcohol should be avoided.

Some women are at increased risk, e.g.

- young mothers: ↑ fetal growth problems; ↑ perinatal morbidity and mortality
- older mothers: Down's syndrome;
- drug abusing women: effects of drugs; HIV; hepatitis B and C.

Ideally, women should be in good health and prepared for pregnancy at the time of conception. The fetus may suffer long-term effects from early adverse influences (Fig. 5.1).

Congenital malformations

About 2% of all babies are born with serious congenital defects, sufficient to threaten life, to cause permanent handicap, or to require surgical correction.

Distressingly little is known of the causes of congenital abnormalities. Single-gene defects and chromosome anomalies account for 10–20% of the total. A small number are attributable to intrauterine infections (e.g.

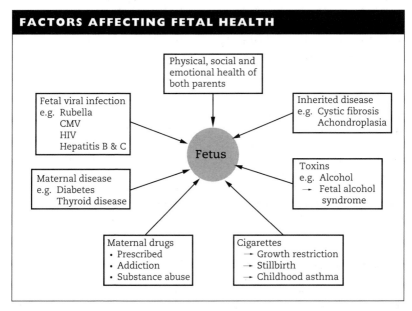

FACTORS AFFECTING FETAL HEALTH

Physical, social and emotional health of both parents

Fetal viral infection
e.g. Rubella
    CMV
    HIV
    Hepatitis B & C

Inherited disease
e.g. Cystic fibrosis
    Achondroplasia

Fetus

Maternal disease
e.g. Diabetes
    Thyroid disease

Toxins
e.g. Alcohol
    → Fetal alcohol
       syndrome

Maternal drugs
• Prescribed
• Addiction
• Substance abuse

Cigarettes
    → Growth restriction
    → Stillbirth
    → Childhood asthma

Fig. 5.1 Factors affecting fetal growth and development.

INCIDENCE OF SOME MAJOR MALFORMATIONS

Down's syndrome	1:600
Club foot	1:700
Polydactyly/syndactyly	1:700
Cleft lip/palate	1:800
Congenital heart disease	1:1000
Spina bifida/anencephaly	1:2000
Oesophageal atresia	1:3000
Diaphragmatic hernia	1:3500

chromosomal anomalies amongst early spontaneous abortuses is very high. Nature has devised a fairly efficient system for terminating at the first possible moment pregnancies that are doomed to failure. It can be shown, for example, that at least 90% of embryos/fetuses with trisomy 21, and a much higher proportion of embryos with sex chromosome anomalies, are aborted. Live-born, malformed infants therefore represent the small minority of abnormal conceptuses.

cytomegalovirus, rubella), fewer to teratogenic drugs and even fewer to ionizing radiation. The ideal is prevention. The paradigm of this is the role of folate in spina bifida. Laboratory and epidemiological studies have confirmed the importance of folate. Increased folate intake has reduced incidence and can prevent recurrence in affected families.

The incidence of serious defects and

Prenatal diagnosis

Choice of technique for prenatal diagnosis is difficult. More invasive tests may provide more definitive information, but may risk precipitation of miscarriage. Amniocentesis has a 1% risk of miscarriage (Table 5.1)

PRENATAL DIAGNOSIS

Mode	Type of investigation	Example
Ultrasound	Fetal measurement	IUGR
	Fetal anomaly	Anencephaly
	Missing structures	Polycystic kidneys
	Enlarged organs	Cardiac
	Abnormalities	Oligohydramnios: IUGR
		Renal agenesis
		Polyhydramnios: oesophageal atresia
Amniocentesis	Fluid analysis	↑ Alphafetoprotein in spina bifida
		↑ Bilirubin in haemolysis
	Fetal cells	Karyotyping/DNA analysis
Maternal blood	Biochemistry	Triple test for Down's syndrome
Chorionic villus sampling	Genetic testing	Karyotyping/DNA analysis
Fetoscopy and fetal blood sampling	Fetal blood and tissue	Wide variety of tests/biopsies

IUGR, intra-uterine growth restriction.

Table 5.1 Modes of prenatal diagnosis.

BENEFITS OF PRENATAL DIAGNOSIS

- Reassurance of parents
- Management of pregnancy and delivery
- Selective termination of pregnancy
- Planned neonatal management
- Possible intrauterine treatment.

Embryonic and fetal growth and development

In early pregnancy the embryological timetable is important in relation to possible teratogenic hazards. Infective, chemical or physical agents that cause birth defects may only be teratogenic at certain times in pregnancy. Rubella, for example, has devastating effects in the first trimester, and almost none in the third trimester.

In the second and third trimesters, fetal growth, estimated clinically or by ultrasound, is an important indicator of fetal health.

The increase in size from conception to birth is phenomenal. At 8 weeks, all major organs have been formed. All serious congenital malformations have their origins in these early weeks. More serious malformations often result in early fetal death and spontaneous abortion.

At 8 weeks the embryo, who only weighs 1 g, becomes a fetus. Weight gain accelerates, and at 6 months (the lower limit of viability) the fetus weighs just over 600 g. Weight gain increases through the final trimester to 100–250 g/week.

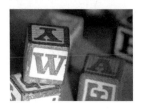

Birth and the Newborn Infant

The delivery of a baby is a wonder. In moments the fetus, crumpled and wet, is transformed into a free-living baby. This transition from intrauterine to extrauterine life is vital. The fetus must escape potential damage during birth, adapt physiologically to adapt to a new environment, and after birth, evade environmental hazards such as hypothermia and infection, to which he is particularly susceptible. The intrapartum and early neonatal period are especially hazardous for the baby who faces intrauterine hypoxia or malnutrition, preterm delivery or major congenital abnormality.

> ⓘ There is a greater risk of dying on the first day of life than on any other day (except the last).

A significant proportion of the population is handicapped in some way by perinatal events. Since almost all of this mortality and morbidity is potentially preventable, the perinatal period offers a unique opportunity to practise effective medicine.

The effects of birth on the fetus

Normal physiology

The most dramatic physiological events related to birth are the switch from placenta to lung as the organ of gas exchange, and the change from fetal to adult circulation that this necessitates.

The right and left sides of the heart are now connected in series rather than in parallel, and the conversion is completed by anatomical closure of the foramen ovale and the ductus arteriosus (p. 130). Most fetuses conduct these events efficiently; a minority suffer potentially damaging asphyxia along the way (Tables 6.1 and 6.2).

Perinatal asphyxia and its prevention

For reasons which are not fully understood the placenta oxygenates fetal blood to a Pao_2 of only about 4 kPa, which equates to the arterial Pao_2 at the summit of Mount Everest. Nevertheless, the oxygen requirements of the fetus are fully met thanks to adaptations such as the high cardiac output (200 mL/kg/min), high haemoglobin concentration (18 g/dL), and the left-shifted

PHYSIOLOGICAL EVENTS AT BIRTH

Phenomena	Effects
Stress of labour $\Rightarrow$ catecholamine and steriod release	$\downarrow$ Lung liquid and $\uparrow$ surfactant release
Uterine contractions $\Rightarrow \downarrow$ placental blood flow	Worsening fetal blood gases
Compression of thorax in birth canal	Expulsion of lung liquid
Thorax recoils on leaving birth canal	Airway fills with air
Clamping of the umbilical cord $\Rightarrow$ hypoxia	Initiation of breathing
$\uparrow$ sensory stimuli (e.g. cold)	Initiation of breathing
Air enters lungs $\Rightarrow \uparrow$ lung tissue oxygen	Pulmonary vascular resistance $\downarrow \Rightarrow$ $\uparrow$ pulmonary blood flow, arterial P_{O_2} and left atrial filling
Low resistance placental circulation stops	Systemic vascular resistance increases
Pressure gradient between atria reverses	Foramen ovale closes functionally
Ductus arteriosus perfused with oxygen-rich blood	Ductus arteriosus closes

Table 6.1 Normal physiological events at birth.

PERINATAL OXYGEN

Requirements	Potential threats
Normal maternal P_{aO_2}	Severe cardiorespiratory disease Hypoxia during anaesthesia
Good uterine blood flow	Maternal vascular disease (e.g. pre-eclampsia, diabetes) Maternal hypotension Prolonged or obstructed labour
Healthy placenta	Placental infarction Placental abruption Intrauterine infection Post-maturity
Good umbilical blood flow	Cord compression during labour Cord prolapse Torn or knotted cord
Normal fetal haemoglobin	Twin-to-twin transfusion Rhesus haemolytic disease
Functioning respiratory centre	Birth asphyxia Respiratory depressant drugs
Patent airway	Position/hypotonia Obstruction by meconium or blood
Healthy heart and lungs	Lung immaturity Diaphragmatic hernia Severe congenital heart disease

Table 6.2 Perinatal oxygen supply.

APGAR SCORE

Score	0	1	2
Heart rate	Absent	<100/min	>100/min or higher
Respiratory effort	None	Slow, irregular	Regular, with cry
Muscle tone	Limp	Some tone in limbs	Active movements
Reflex irritability	None	Grimace only	Cry
Colour	Pallor	Body blue	Pink all over

Table 6.3 Apgar score, usually recorded at 1, 5 and 10 minutes after birth.

dissociation curve of fetal haemoglobin (HbF) which allows greater oxygen saturation of haemoglobin at a given Pa_{O_2} (p. 202). The fetus sits on the steep part of the dissociation curve so that only a small drop in Pa_{O_2} will result in a large reduction in blood oxygen content. As a result, oxygenation around the time of birth is in a state of delicate balance which depends critically on many factors.

It is not surprising that the fetus has evolved defences against acute hypoxia. These include redistribution of blood flow in favour of vital tissues, and a myocardium and nervous system better able to withstand hypoxia than the adult. A small minority of fetuses, however, suffer perinatal brain damage. Hypoxia therefore calls for prompt obstetric action and resuscitation at birth in order to prevent progression.

Resuscitation

Rapid assessment and action is needed for any baby who does not breathe within 30 s of birth, or who exhibits slow or irregular gasping. Bradycardia indicates hypoxia (Table 6.3). In almost all infants, adequate ventilation and oxygenation will be all that is needed for effective resuscitation. Simple actions done well prevent mortality and morbidity.

Risk of hypothermia is reduced by drying and use of a radiant heat source (Fig. 6.1). First the mouth, and then the nose are

POINTERS TO HYPOXIA

Antepartum
- intrauterine growth retardation
- reduced fetal movements
- abnormal fetal bloodflow (Dopplers)

Intrapartum
- meconium-stained liquor
- abnormal fetal heart rate (cardiotocograph)
- metabolic acidosis (fetal blood sample)

Postpartum
- bradycardia/apnoea
- low Apgar score
- delayed onset of respiration
- metabolic acidosis (cord blood)

cleared of secretions with a soft suction catheter. In the correct position, the neck is extended allowing for the infant's large occiput. If hypoxia is not far advanced, breathing can usually be started by stimulation: rubbing with a towel that has been through an NHS laundry dries and stimulates! If there is no response, or the heart rate is below 100, or the baby is pale, limp and immobile, intermittent positive pressure ventilation is begun either by bag and mask or by an endotracheal tube.

Infants who make a rapid recovery should be given to their mothers as soon as possible. Only severely asphyxiated babies

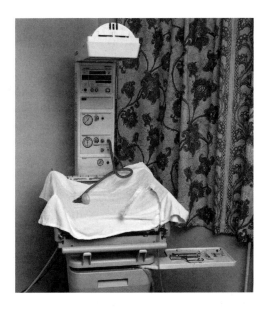

Fig. 6.1 The resuscitaire comprises a heater, source of oxygen and suction, and an equipped platform for neonatal resuscitation.

need be admitted to a special care baby unit for further care.

Birth asphyxia

Birth asphyxia is the consequence of intrapartum hypoxia when the baby needs advanced resuscitation and goes on to have an *hypoxic ischaemic encephalopathy (HIE)*. HIE occurs in 1–2 per 1000 deliveries.

The baby who is delivered after severe intrapartum hypoxia has a characteristic clinical picture. He is bradycardic, pale, limp and apnoeic and has a severe metabolic acidosis, accumulated during a period of anaerobic glycolysis. Prompt resuscitation is important.

HIE is graded by severity.
• *Mild*: irritability and abnormal handling, a high pitched cry and poor feeding.
• *Moderate*: lethargy and initial hypotonia, decreased spontaneous movements, poor feeding and occasional fits.
• *Severe*: diminished conscious level, no spontaneous movement, multiple seizures which are difficult to control, and multi-organ failure.

HIE requires intensive care. Infants in the severe group have a >70% risk of cerebral damage. It is estimated that 15–30% of cerebral palsy is secondary to intrapartum hypoxic ischaemic damage.

Routine care of the normal baby

Vitamin K. Newborn babies have low levels of vitamin K and its dependent clotting factors, and some of them will bleed from the gastrointestinal tract, into the skin or mucous membranes, or rarely into the brain. Haemorrhagic disease is limited to infants who have not received prophylaxis. Vitamin K is given as an oral supplement or as a single IM injection. Oral vitamin K is repeated over the first month in breast-fed infants.

The umbilical cord has two arteries and one vein. A single artery may be associated with congenital malformation. The cord is clamped about 1 cm from the skin surface and cut close to the clamp. Most units use some form of antiseptic preparation on the cord stump until it has separated, which is usually by about one week. The cord should be observed carefully for signs of infection.

Labelling. All newborn babies should have name bands attached to wrist and ankle in the delivery room and in the presence of the mother.

Bathing. It is tempting to wash the newborn clean after birth, but bathing carries a serious risk of cooling and can be deferred for a few days. Vernix, a natural layer of grease which is present *in utero*, is absorbed naturally.

Passage of meconium and urine. It is important to note the time of first passing meconium and urine. Sometimes this occurs at or soon after delivery, but both are usually passed within 24 h of birth. Delay in bowel or bladder function should prompt a search for underlying pathology.

Feeding. This topic is dealt with fully in Chapter 8 (p. 75). There is much to be said for putting the baby to the breast shortly after birth. The first feed, of either breast milk or a formula, should be offered within 3–6 h of birth.

Examination of the newborn

All newborn babies should have a clinical examination within the first 24 h of life. Unless there is a good reason, the mother should be present, and in the vast majority, the doctor will be able to reassure parents that all is well. The aims of newborn examinations are to:
• Detect conditions that:
  ♦ will benefit from early treatment, e.g. congenital dislocation of the hip
  ♦ need long-term supervision, e.g. congenital heart disease, club foot
  ♦ have genetic implications, e.g. Down's syndrome

  ♦ indicate systemic illness, e.g. congenital pneumonia.
• Discuss parental anxieties, and to take a brief medical, genetic and social history, seeking information that may be relevant to the future health and development of the baby.
• Provide advice on matters such as infant feeding, attendance at baby clinics, and immunization.
• Advise on minor abnormalities which may lead to worry.

Suggested scheme for routine clinical examination

General observation. Does the infant look well? Is she pink and wriggly? Is she tachypnoeic or pale? Check for the normal flexed posture and symmetrical limb movements. Are there dysmorphic features? Look for cyanosis, jaundice, skin rashes and birth marks.

Measurements. Weight, length and occipito-frontal head circumference are evaluated for gestational age by reference to a centile chart.

Head. Check head shape, allowing for moulding that occurs during birth, and assess the tension of the anterior fontanelle and the width of the sutures. If the fontanelle feels unusually full or if there is more than 1 cm of sutural separation, hydrocephalus should be suspected and ultrasound examination performed.

Face. Look for signs of facial nerve palsy and dysmorphic features.

Eyes. Asymmetry of eye size is abnormal: one eye may be small (congenital infection or developmental defect) or the other eye may be large (congenital glaucoma). The eye should be checked for signs of infection. The red reflex excludes cataract.

COMMON CONDITIONS OF LITTLE CLINICAL IMPORTANCE

- Skin lesions
  - Strawberry naevi (p. 181)
  - 'Stork' marks (p. 181)
  - Milia (Small collections in the sebaceous glands which disappear soon after birth.) (Fig. 6.2)
  - Urticaria neonatorum (A blotchy red rash; each spot has a yellow centre which is full of eosinophils. Individual spots come and go. It is benign and should be distinguished from skin sepsis.)
  - Mongolian blue spots (p. 182)
  - Epithelial 'pearls' (Small white cysts near the midline on the palate.)

- Subconjunctive haemorrhage

- Cephalhaematoma (p. 62)

- Positional talipes (p. 174)

- Peripheral and traumatic cyanosis (Blue hands and feet are normal in the first days. Facial congestion may at first look like cyanosis.)

- Breast enlargement

- Oral and vulval mucosal tags

- Sacral dimple (Extremely rarely connects with spinal cord.)

- Skin tags and diminutive accessory digits

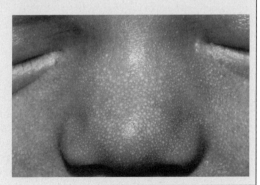

Fig. 6.2 Milia. Small raised, white spots over the nose and cheeks.

Nose. The nose is the baby's principal airway and should be checked for signs of obstruction.

Mouth. A baby will usually open its mouth if gentle downward pressure is applied to the chin. The palate should be inspected for clefts and palpated for submucosal clefts (Fig. 6.3). The oral cavity should be checked for the presence of teeth, cysts or thrush (candida infection).

PRIMITIVE REFLEXES

- Grasp—hands and feet—birth to 4 months

- Moro—startle reflex—birth to 4 months
  - hold the infant supporting the head, and allow the head to drop a few centimetres. The infant will look surprised, throw its arms outwards and then bring them back to the midline.

- Asymmetric tonic neck reflex (ATNR)—birth to 7 months
  - on turning the head to one side, the ipsilateral arm and leg are extended.

- Rooting reflex—from birth
  - on touching the infant's face, he turns, opening his mouth as if to suck on the finger.

Persistence of the Moro and ATNR is abnormal and may indicate cerebral palsy

Jaw. A small or recessed mandible (retrognathia) can lead to feeding difficulty or respiratory obstruction.

Chest. Check the baby is pink and not breathless.

Heart. Note the side of the chest on which the apex is felt, and the forcefulness of the cardiac impulse. Heart murmurs at this age are very common and relate to the transition from fetal to adult circulatory pattern. It is difficult even for experienced cardiologists to distinguish clinically significant murmurs from non-significant ones. It is important, however, not to generate widespread parental anxiety. A few days later, many transitional murmurs will have disappeared. As a rule, soft, mid or early systolic murmurs are likely to be insignificant, whereas pansystolic, diastolic, or very loud murmurs are likely to be important.

Abdomen. The liver edge is usually palpable 1–2 cm below the right costal margin and the spleen can be tipped in at least 20% of normal babies. The lower poles of both kidneys may be palpable.

Groins. Ensure that both femoral pulses can be felt, as their absence may denote coarctation of the aorta. Check for hernias.

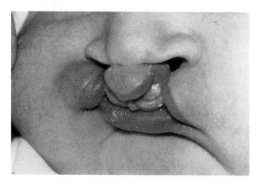

Fig. 6.3 Bilateral cleft lip and palate.

Genitalia. Check that the genitalia are clearly either male or female. If there is doubt, do not ascribe sex. In boys, check that the testes are in the scrotum and that the urethral meatus is where it should be. In girls, inspect the genitalia and remember that a little vaginal bleeding or discharge of clear mucus is normal secondary to the influence of maternal and placental hormones.

Anus. Ask if the baby has passed meconium, and check that the anus is present and normally located.

Spine. Turn the baby prone and look for scoliosis. The entire dorsal midline should be inspected for lumps, naevi, hairy patches, pits or sinuses which may indicate spinal cord abnormality.

Hips. Examination of the hips is very important (p. 179). It is best left to the end of the examination as it may upset the baby.

Central nervous system. A full neurological assessment of the newborn is time-consuming and demands considerable skill and experience. Observe the spontaneously moving baby while conducting the rest of the examination, looking for symmetry. Ask about feeding behaviour. Assess tone by picking the baby up and holding her in ventral suspension. Elicit the Moro reflex (p. 60).

Biochemical screening. Routine screening on blood-spot tests is carried out on day 5–7 for phenylketonuria (p. 215) (Guthrie test) and hypothyroidism (p. 213). Some hospitals also screen for cystic fibrosis.

Birth injury (physical trauma)

In a modern obstetric unit serious birth injury, such as tearing of the dura or spinal cord is rare, but evidence of lesser degrees of trauma is quite commonly discovered on routine examination. Trauma is predisposed to by factors such as obstructed labour (due to small pelvis or large baby), precipitate labour, malpresentation and heroic instrumental delivery.

Nerve palsies

Most lesions recover as traumatic swelling subsides, but minor disability persists in about 15% and a few are left handicapped.

Brachial plexus palsy

These are associated with large fetal size and difficult delivery. *Erb's palsy* affects C5/6 roots, resulting in weakness or paralysis. The affected arm lies straight and limp beside the trunk, internally rotated and with the fingers flexed (waiter's tip position). When the Moro reflex is elicited, the affected arm does not respond. Less commonly the lower roots C8/T1 are injured resulting in weakness of wrist extensors and intrinsic muscles of the hand (*Klumpke's palsy*).

Facial nerve palsy

The facial nerve may be injured by pressure from the maternal pelvic bones or by forceps blades. It is a lower motor neurone defect, usually unilateral.

Phrenic nerve palsy

Infrequently, the cervical roots of the phrenic nerve are damaged causing diaphragmatic paralysis and respiratory difficulty.

Skeletal injury

Clavicle fracture

This commonly follows shoulder dystocia. Complete breaks are painful and limit the baby's arm movements. Clavicle fractures heal well, but often with considerable callus formation.

Humerus and femur
Fractures and epiphyseal injury may occur during difficult births. They heal well.

Skull fractures
The compliant skull of the newborn is remarkably resistant to fracture. Asymptomatic linear fractures of the parietal bone

are commonest. Depressed fractures require surgical elevation.

Soft tissue injuries

Cephalhaematoma
Subperiosteal bleeding occurs in 1–2%, usually over the parietal bone. The extent of the swelling, and therefore the amount of blood loss, is limited by the attachment of the periosteum to the margins of each skull bone (Fig. 6.4). The vast majority resolve spontaneously, although the edge of the lesion may calcify.

Subaponeurotic haemorrhage
Haemorrhage between the periosteum and galea aponeurotica is not limited in the same way as a cephalhaematoma, and serious blood loss can occur. It is more common after ventouse delivery. The baby appears pale with a raised fluctuant swelling of the scalp.

Sternomastoid tumour
This is a fusiform fibrous mass in the middle of the sternomastoid muscle. It may follow trauma. It usually disappears over about 6 months. Gentle physiotherapy to prevent shortening of the muscle is required.

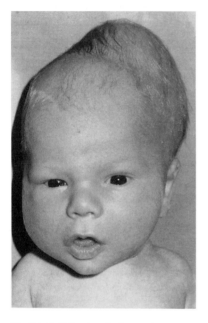

Fig. 6.4 Unilateral cephalhaematoma.

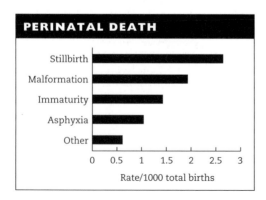

Fig. 6.5 Causes of perinatal death (the stillbirth rate is for fetuses without abnormality).

Bruising and abrasions

Difficult births are often accompanied by bruising. Usually there is little serious harm. Breakdown of extravasated blood may contribute to neonatal jaundice. Skin abrasions are portals of entry for microorganisms and should be observed for signs of infection.

Congenital malformations

Of all the causes of perinatal death, congenital abnormalities have shown the least decline over the years (Fig. 6.5). Most of the common defects are described in the relevant chapter. Causation and prenatal diagnosis are discussed in Chapter 5 (p. 50).

At birth, most congenital defects can be detected by the routine clinical examination or will present symptoms such as vomiting, cyanosis, jaundice or failure to pass urine or meconium. Some abnormalities, especially in the cardiovascular system or renal tract, may escape detection. It is important to remember that multiple defects are quite common and finding of any anomaly should always lead to a careful search for others. Constellations of defects may fit into recognized syndromes and every effort should be made to arrive at a diagnosis in these cases, as it may be possible to give a reasonably accurate prognosis and genetic risk of recurrence.

The problems of helping parents to cope with the bad news that there is something wrong with their baby are discussed in Chapter 2.

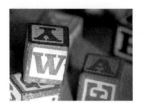

Disorders of the Newborn

Definitions

• Low birthweight (LBW) — 2500 g or less (7% of UK births)
• Very low birthweight (VLBW) — 1500 g or less (1% of UK births)
• Extremely low birthweight — 1000 g or less
• Preterm — less than 37 completed weeks gestation (6% of UK births) (two-thirds of LBW babies are preterm)
• Term — 37–41 weeks gestation
• Post-term — 42 weeks or more
• Small for gestational age (SGA): birthweight below 3rd centile for sex and gestation
• Large for gestational age: birthweight above 97th centile for sex and gestation
• Appropriate for gestational age (AGA): birthweight between 3rd and 97th centiles for sex and gestation.

The correct classification of a baby by weight and gestation is important (Fig. 7.1). Abnormalities of weight for gestation may indicate maternal diabetes, intrauterine infection or chromosome abnormality. The clinical problems of the preterm infant are due to immaturity. Light-for-dates babies are at risk of hypoglycaemia (p. 68).

The best guide to gestation is the menstrual history combined with an ultrasound estimate of fetal size made before 20 weeks' gestation. Physical and neurological features of the newborn give a rough estimate of gestation. With increasing gestation, skin becomes keratinized, thicker, and has less lanugo (fine hair). Ear cartilage and the breast nodule develop during the third trimester. In boys, the testes descend into the scrotum around 36 weeks. In girls, the labia majora cover the labia minora towards term. As gestation increases, muscle tone and ligamentous laxity increase.

The preterm baby

Principal problems are due to immaturity:
• respiratory distress syndrome (surfactant deficiency)
• recurrent apnoea
• poor thermoregulation
• renal function, fluid and electrolyte balance
• nutrition
• patent ductus arteriosus
• intraventricular haemorrhage and other CNS damage
• anaemia
• necrotizing enterocolilitis
• jaundice.

GROWTH CHART

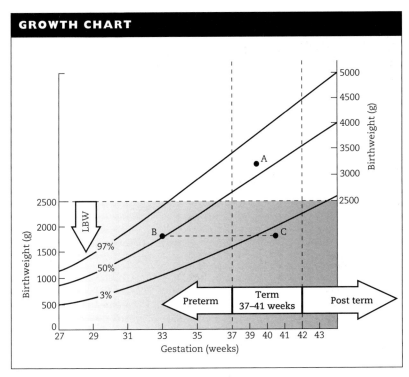

Fig. 7.1 Growth chart with 50th, 3rd and 97th centiles. Three babies are marked: A is term and appropriate for gestation; B and C both have the same birthweight and both are LBW but they will have very different clinical problems; B is LBW and preterm—he is appropriate for gestation; C is LBW and term—he is small for gestation.

Respiratory distress syndrome (RDS)

RDS, also known as *hyaline membrane disease*, is virtually confined to preterm babies and is the most serious of the problems.

> **i** Antenatal maternal steroids lead to a 60% reduction in the likelihood of RDS, and should be used whenever possible.

Pulmonary surfactant lowers surface tension at the interface between inspired gas and the liquid that lines the respiratory tract. Without surfactant the alveoli cannot

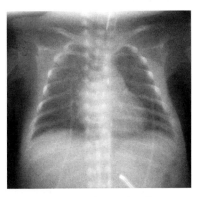

Fig. 7.2 Chest X-ray in RDS showing granularity and air bronchograms.

be inflated and tend to collapse. Structural immaturity of the lungs and chest wall and poor respiratory drive add to the problem. The end result is atelectasis, which disturbs gas exchange, and gives rise to the appearance shown in the X-ray (Fig. 7.2). Increased work of breathing, which, if it cannot be sustained, leads to carbon dioxide retention and often to apnoeic spells.

SIGNS OF RESPIRATORY DISTRESS

- Tachypnoea (>60 bpm)
- Intercostals recession
- Subcostal recession
- Grunting
- Nasal flare
- Cyanosis

The natural history of RDS is resolution over a period of 3–7 days as surfactant production increases, and the management is to keep the baby alive and undamaged during this period. The mainstay of management is some form of assisted ventilation. Surfactant replacement therapy is given through the endotracheal tube soon after birth, and leads to reduced mortality, less risk of pneumothorax and reduced lung damage. Careful monitoring is crucial. An essential part of therapy is stability of blood gas status (homeostasis): low oxygen is damaging; high oxygen may lead to retinopathy of prematurity; high carbon dioxide predisposes to brain haemorrhage; low levels increase risk of ischaemic brain lesions.

Bronchopulmonary dysplasia (BPD)

This chronic lung disease occurs in some preterm babies who have been ventilated for severe RDS. It is due to lung damage by high oxygen concentration and high positive pressures. Steroid therapy is helpful, but some babies with BPD require prolonged oxygen therapy.

Temperature control

Hypothermia increases oxygen consumption and predisposes to RDS and infection. It must be avoided. Incubators and radiant heaters are used so that the baby uses little energy keeping warm or cooling down.

RISK FACTORS FOR HYPOTHERMIA

- Large surface area relative to body mass
- Little subcutaneous fat
- Large insensible water and heat loss

Fluid and electrolyte balance

Renal function is relatively poor in the preterm baby. Coupled with a high but largely unmeasurable water loss through the very permeable skin, this can lead rapidly to dehydration and electrolyte disturbance.

Nutrition

If the preterm newborn is to equal the fetal growth rate, requirements are high (Table 7.1).

If the baby is in good health, milk is given. Nutritive sucking and swallowing develops at about 34 weeks. Frequent, small volume gastric feeds are used. The milk of choice is the mother's expressed breast milk—it is better tolerated, induces gut maturation, and reduces risk of necrotizing enterocolitis. In VLBW infants, protein and calories are added to breast milk. For tiny sick babies, parenteral nutrition is often used.

PRETERM NUTRITION

Energy	120 calories/kg/day
Water	150–180 ml/kg/day
Protein	3.5 g/kg/day
Fat	6 g/kg/day
Glucose	12 g/kg/day

Table 7.1 Preterm nutritional requirements.

Patent ductus arteriosus (PDA)

The ductus arteriosus of the preterm infant often fails to close, especially when RDS is present. Left-to-right shunting may lead to heart failure. The PDA can be closed by giving a prostaglandin synthetase inhibitor (e.g. indomethacin), but sometimes surgical closure is required.

Intraventricular haemorrhage and other forms of brain damage

In the walls of the lateral ventricles of preterm babies are fragile capillaries, where bleeding may occur during hypoxia or RDS. Haemorrhage, which is demonstrated by cranial ultrasound, may be local or extend into the ventricles or cerebral tissue. The more extensive the haemorrhage, the more likely are brain damage and hydrocephalus. It is estimated that some degree of haemorrhage occurs in 40% of very small babies, although it causes serious damage in only a small minority.

In the brain of the preterm infant, the periventricular white matter is prone to ischaemic injury (*periventricular leukomalacia*), characteristically leading to spastic diplegia.

Anaemia

In babies of all gestations, haemoglobin concentration falls from the high level appropriate to fetal life. In the preterm baby, this fall is more pronounced and exacerbated by multiple blood tests. Early anaemia is not due to a deficiency of haematinics and cannot be prevented by iron supplementation. A *late* anaemia may occur and most preterm infants are given iron supplementation from 6 weeks of age.

Necrotizing enterocolitis (NEC)

NEC is the commonest surgical emergency in neonatal medicine. Surgery is often needed. Mortality is 20%. It is almost restricted to the preterm. Aetiology is unknown, but immaturity, infection, gut ischaemia, and enteral milk feeding all contribute to pathogenesis.

Management of the preterm infant

Preterm infants who are unwell are looked after in neonatal units or special care baby units (SCBU) (Fig. 7.3).

Admission criteria to these units should be strict so that as few babies as possible are separated from their mothers. Parents must be allowed free access to their baby while on SCBU and every effort must be made to involve them in their baby's care as much as possible. Hospitals that cannot provide long-term intensive care often transfer infants to a Regional Unit where such facilities exist. Babies travel quite well in expert hands.

As a result of growing experience in the techniques of mechanical ventilation and supportive care, the mortality rate among preterm infants has fallen considerably and continues to do so. The survival rate for babies of less than 1500 g birthweight who

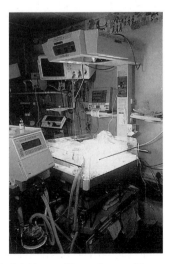

Fig. 7.3 Neonatal intensive care. The hi-tech set-up is daunting for the parents.

SGA BABIES

Type	Growth pattern	Causes
Asymmetrical	Head circumference significantly higher on centiles than on weight	Late fetal malnutrition Pre-eclampsia Smoking
Symmetrical	Head circumference and weight equally reduced	Genetic Normal small Fetal abnormality Early fetal malnutrition Congenital viral infection Drug effect

Table 7.2 Types of SGA baby.

are free of lethal malformation is currently better than 80%. This increased survival has yet to be fully evaluated in terms of quality but serious handicap occurs in no more than 6–10%. Survival rates fall off rapidly at gestations below 26 weeks.

The small-for-gestational-age (SGA) baby

PROBLEMS OF THE SGA INFANT

- Perinatal asphyxia
  - Poor placental function
  - Risk of meconium aspiration (especially in post term)

- Hypoglycaemia (especially asymmetric)

- Congenital malformation or chromosome abnormality (especially symmetric)

- Poor postnatal growth (especially symmetric)

- Hypothermia

Paediatric management begins by anticipating delivery. The SGA infant is more likely to need resuscitation and the paediatrician will be needed if meconium is present in the liquor to prevent aspiration. Small size and little insulation from body fat increases risk of hypothermia (Fig. 7.4). The most important, common problem is hypoglycaemia (p. 71). This should be anticipated with early, frequent feeds and routine surveillance of blood sugar, while staying alert to hypoglycaemic symptoms.

Most SGA infants, especially those with late placental insufficiency and asymmetric intrauterine growth restriction (Table 7.2), have a good prognosis. SGA infants, however, are at increased risk of neurodevelopmental impairment. Growth retardation evident before 20 weeks' gestation affects brain growth as well as somatic growth, and these babies often fail to show 'catch up' growth postnatally.

Respiratory problems in the term infant

Respiratory symptoms in the newborn are not always due to primary lung disorder. Brain damage, metabolic acidosis, congenital heart disease, disorders of the

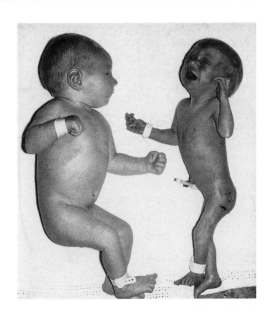

Fig. 7.4 Two babies born at term. The baby on the right shows severe growth restriction.

diaphragm such as phrenic nerve palsy or muscle hypoplasia, and space-occupying lesions within the thorax such as pneumothorax, pleural effusion or diaphragmatic hernia, can lead to respiratory distress. The following lung disorders are common:

Transient tachypnoea. Tachypnoea for a few hours after birth due to delayed clearance of lung fluid. It is more common after caesarean section.

Meconium aspiration. Intrapartum asphyxia in full-term babies may cause passage of meconium into the liquor. If inhaled, it can cause airway obstruction and pneumonitis. Clearing the upper airway and trachea of meconium at birth has reduced the incidence of this serious condition.

Congenital pneumonia. When microorganisms invade the amniotic cavity before delivery the baby may be born with an established pneumonia. This is particularly likely when there has been prolonged rupture of the membranes (longer than 24 h). Group B streptococci (GBS) and Gram-negative organisms such as *Escherichia coli* are most commonly incriminated.

Pneumothorax. Tiny, spontaneous pneumothoraces are not uncommon after birth and they are usually asymptomatic. Occasionally they produce symptoms, and very occasionally, a chest drain is necessary.

Jaundice

Around 50% of infants are visibly jaundiced during the first week of life. The commonest mechanism is described as 'physiological' and reflects a temporary inadequacy in the system of conjugation. In the fetus, very little conjugation of bilirubin is desirable, but after birth conjugation and hepatic excretion of bilirubin must take over from placental transfer.

It is important to recognize infants who

do not need investigation or intervention, other than to measure the bilirubin level if clinically indicated. These infants obey the 'golden rules of physiological jaundice':

- jaundice not apparent in first 24 h
- the infant remains well
- the serum bilirubin does not reach treatment level
- the jaundice has faded by 14 days.

> Jaundice apparent with the first 24 h is never physiological and strongly suggests excessive haemolysis or sepsis.

Kernicterus

Unconjugated bilirubin (but not conjugated) can enter the nervous system and cause neuronal damage. High serum biliru-bin, preterm birth, acidosis or hypoxia increases risk. Bilirubin is normally bound to albumin so that hypoalbuminaemia and drugs that displace bilirubin from albumin should be avoided.

The rare clinical syndrome of bilirubin encephalopathy (*kernicterus*) may result in death or serious handicap. When serum bilirubin is high, treatment with phototherapy is started. Phototherapy uses light of a wavelength that converts unconjugated bilirubin to non-toxic isomers which can be excreted without conjugation. Phototherapy takes time to work; if a rapid fall in bilirubin is required an exchange transfusion must be performed (Fig. 7.5).

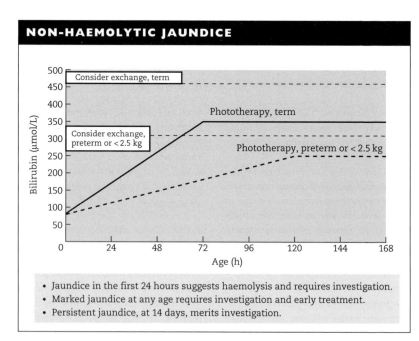

NON-HAEMOLYTIC JAUNDICE

Consider exchange, term

Phototherapy, term

Consider exchange, preterm or < 2.5 kg

Phototherapy, preterm or < 2.5 kg

Bilirubin (µmol/L)

Age (h)

- Jaundice in the first 24 hours suggests haemolysis and requires investigation.
- Marked jaundice at any age requires investigation and early treatment.
- Persistent jaundice, at 14 days, merits investigation.

Fig. 7.5 Serum bilirubin is plotted against age to decide upon therapy.

CAUSES OF NEONATAL JAUNDICE

- Physiological

- Haemolytic (often begins < 24 h)
  - ABO incompatibility
  - Rhesus isoimmunization
  - Other isoimmunization (e.g. Kell, c)
  - Red cell defects (e.g. spherocytosis, G6PD deficiency)

- Physiological plus
  - Prematurity
  - Bruising
  - Polycythaemia
  - Dehydration
  - Sepsis
  - Gut obstruction

- Prolonged
  - Physiological (for those who have not read textbooks!)
  - Breast milk
  - Neonatal hepatitis
  - Hypothyroidism
  - Inborn errors of metabolism (e.g. galactosaemia)
  - Abnormal biliary tract (e.g. biliary atresia)

Pathological jaundice

If haemolysis is suspected, look for maternal antibodies and check the baby's bilirubin, haemoglobin and Coombs' test.

ABO incompatibility is the commonest cause of haemolytic jaundice, and usually occurs in a group A baby of a group O mother. It occasionally requires an exchange transfusion. Rhesus haemolytic disease used to be the commonest cause of serious haemolysis, capable of causing profound jaundice and anaemia, but it is now rare because of the use of anti-D immunoglobulin.

Breast milk jaundice is quite common, usually presenting as delayed resolution of physiological jaundice. Precise mechanisms are debated, but the milk of some mothers seems to interfere with conjugation. If clinical and biochemical investigation is satisfactory, breast feeding can continue.

> **i** Biliary atresia is rare, but early recognition is essential for successful surgery. The cardinal features are prolonged conjugated jaundice and pale stools. It must be considered in all babies who are still jaundiced at 14 days.

Hypoglycaemia

HIGH RISK OF HYPOGLYCAEMIA

- Small for gestatational age
- Preterm
- Polycythaemia
- Post asphyxia
- Infants of diabetic mothers

At birth, the plentiful supplies of glucose that cross the placenta are cut off and the baby must maintain her own blood sugar from stored glycogen and fat until feeding is established. Glucose is an essential fuel for the nervous system, and hypoglycaemia, with symptoms of irritability, pallor, reluctance to feed and, most severely, seizures, rapidly leads to neuronal damage. The danger level for blood sugar is in the region of 1–1.5 mmol/L. Such levels have been found in healthy asymptomatic term infants, in whom the brain is protected by its ability to use other fuels. In infants from high risk groups, and in those with symptoms, it is essential to keep blood glucose at or above 2.5 mmol/L, by early and frequent milk feeds and, if necessary, by i.v. infusion of dextrose. In these infants, blood sugar is checked 4–6 hourly until the risk of hypoglycaemia is passed.

Infant of a diabetic mother

If a mother has a diabetes or gestational diabetes, the altered metabolic climate of the fetus can cause the following problems:

- hypoglycaemia
- large size and obesity
- increased risk of RDS
- polycythaemia
- congenital malformation.

Good diabetic control before conception and during pregnancy can greatly reduce these problems.

Hypocalcaemia

Hypocalcaemia (i.e. serum calcium below 1.7 mmol/L) may cause apnoea, neuromuscular excitability or seizures. It is most likely to arise in preterm infants, infants of diabetic mothers and following birth asphyxia. Hypocalcaemic seizures, unlike those of hypoglycaemia, have a good prognosis.

Infection

Fetal infection

Micro-organisms rarely succeed in crossing the placenta or penetrating the intact amnion. The effect of fetal infection depends on the nature of the organism, and the stage of gestation. Very early infections may cause fetal death, abortion or major malformation.

Rubella. The rubella virus causes malformation if infection occurs early in pregnancy. An infected baby may also be born with evidence of active viraemia as shown by jaundice, hepatosplenomegaly, purpura and sometimes lesions of the bones and lungs (Fig. 7.6). This may follow infection later in pregnancy and not lead to malformation.

Cytomegalovirus (CMV). The incidence of congenital CMV infection is in the region of

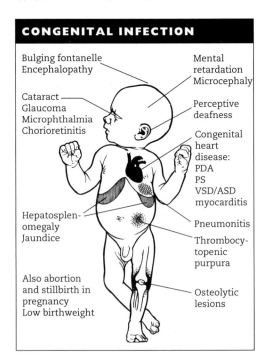

CONGENITAL INFECTION

Bulging fontanelle
Encephalopathy

Cataract
Glaucoma
Microphthalmia
Chorioretinitis

Hepatosplen-
omegaly
Jaundice

Also abortion
and stillbirth in
pregnancy
Low birthweight

Mental
retardation
Microcephaly

Perceptive
deafness

Congenital
heart
disease:
PDA
PS
VSD/ASD
myocarditis

Pneumonitis

Thrombocy-
topenic
purpura

Osteolytic
lesions

Fig. 7.6 Features of congenital rubella syndrome.

3 or 4 cases per 1000 births. The brain and auditory pathway are the major targets for damage, which occurs in about 15% of infected fetuses.

Toxoplasmosis. This rare disease is caused by a protozoon whose usual host is the cat. CNS involvement with hydrocephalus and chorioretinitis may occur.

Human immunodeficiency virus (HIV) (p. 227). Approximately 10–20% of infants of HIV seropositive mothers are prenatally or perinatally infected with HIV. This vertical transmission presently accounts for the majority of AIDS in childhood. Symptoms of AIDS may begin at any time from birth, and usually within 2 years. Commoner symptoms are failure to thrive, diarrhoea, recurrent infections, and severe candida infection. The number of AIDS cases in babies and young children in the UK is small. Worldwide it is rapidly becoming the major cause of infant mortality.

Vertical transmission of HIV is reduced by:
- antenatal, maternal antiviral therapy
- delivery by caesarean section
- avoidance of breast feeding.

Hepatitis B infection. Risk of vertical transmission varies, but is high if mothers have the e antigen. Such babies are protected by a combination of passive immunity with hepatitis B immune globulin and active immunity with hepatitis B vaccine. Lower risk babies should receive hepatitis B vaccine.

Syphilis, tuberculosis and malaria can cause fetal infection; all three are rare in the UK.

Intrapartum infection

When the membranes rupture the fetus may be invaded by the flora of the birth canal. The following infections are particularly likely to be acquired in this way:
- Pneumonia and/or meningitis due to group B streptococci or *Listeria monocytogenes*
- Gonoccocal ophthalmia
- *Candida albicans*
- *Herpes simplex.*

Infection acquired after birth

Once born, the baby rapidly becomes colonized by bacteria and usually this occurs without harm. Infection is especially likely if colonization is heavy or if the organisms are of high pathogenicity. Organisms in the blood stream may give rise to septicaemia, meningitis or pneumonia.

> ### COMMON EARLY SIGNS OF SEPSIS
>
> - Lethargy and hypotonia
> - Poor feeding, abdominal distension or vomiting
> - Pallor and mottling of the skin
> - Disturbed temperature regulation
> - Recurrent apnoea

Any baby suspected of being infected should be examined carefully and investigated promptly with blood culture, chest X-ray, microscopy and culture of urine and CSF. Broad-spectrum antibiotic therapy is started pending results. *Group B Streptococcus* infection is a dangerous, rapidly progressive infection, which must be suspected in an infant who has suggestive symptoms. Immediate investigation and antibiotic may be life saving. Other common organisms causing serious infection are *E. coli, Staphylococcus aureus*, and Listeria. Coagulase negative staphylococcus is the commonest pathogen in the preterm.

Sticky eye

The cause of most sticky eyes is poor drainage down the nasolacrimal duct.

Often all that is necessary is to bathe the eye with warm saline. More serious eye infections may be due to staphylococci and coliforms. Occasionally *Chlamydia trachomatis* and gonococcus cause severe purulent eye infection in the first 10 days and need urgent diagnosis and treatment.

Skin infection

Septic spots and paronychia, usually due to staphylococcal infection, are relatively common and responsive to local treatment, but may need systemic antibiotics.

Candida infection

Infection of the mouth and nappy area by yeasts is common. It responds well to nystatin or miconazole. Therapy should be continued for a few days longer than it takes to clear the signs of infection. Hygiene of bottles and dummies must be scrupulous.

Convulsions

Convulsions occurring in the first 48 h of life are usually due to intrapartum brain damage and are generally a bad prognostic sign. Other causes of seizures are meningitis, hypoglycaemia, hypocalcaemia, hypomagnesaemia, hypo- or hypernatraemia, and inborn errors of metabolism.

Seizures always require immediate and thorough investigation and treatment of any underlying disorder. If the cause cannot be remedied, anticonvulsant medication is given.

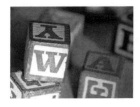

Nutrition

Infant and child nutrition is the foundation stone of healthy growth which in turn facilitates healthy development. Worldwide, the only common nutritional problem is starvation. In industrialized societies the main problems are eating unwisely or eating too much. In clinical practice, nutritional care is central to the management of all chronic diseases.

Nutrition is particularly important in the first year of life, when the infant is entirely dependent on his carers to feed him. Babies treble their birth weight in the first year of life; to treble it again takes 10 years. Furthermore, 65% of total postnatal brain growth takes place in the first year of life. Starvation may permanently hamper both physical and mental development.

> **ⓘ** Fetal and infant nutrition determines risk of adult cardiovascular disease and diabetes—an example of nutritional programming

Infant nutrition

Milk

Milk is a rich source of energy, proteins and minerals. It is the sole source of nutrition for the first months, and provides an essential part of energy, protein and calcium intake in pre-school children. Cow's milk has a high mineral content and osmolality. Infant formula feeds are modified to approximate their content to that of breast milk.

Unmodified cow's milk should not be given before 6 months of age, and most recommend breast or formula feeding to 12 months. As a rule, children should drink whole milk, and not fat reduced. Cow's milk contains inadequate amounts of vitamins and iron, and supplements are needed in infancy unless a full mixed solid diet has been achieved.

AVERAGE REQUIREMENTS IN INFANCY	
Water	150 mL/kg/day
Calories	110 kcal/kg/day
Vitamin C	15 mg/day
Vitamin D	400 i.u./day
Calcium	600 mg/day
Iron	6 mg/day

NUTRITIONAL CONTENT OF MILK

	Human milk	Cow's milk	Infant formula
Energy (kCal)	68	64	66
Protein (g)	1.3	3.1	1.4
Casein	32%	77%	40%
Whey	68%	23%	60%
Lactose (g)	7.0	4.8	7.0
Fat (g)	3.7	3.7	3.6
Saturated	48%	58%	41%
Sodium (mmol)	0.7	2.5	0.8
Calcium (mmol)	0.9	2.8	1.3
Phosphorus (mmol)	0.4	2.5	0.7
Iron (mg)	0.08	0.06	0.50

Table 8.1 Nutritional content of three different types of milk per 100 mL (100 mL = 3.5 fluid ounces).

Breast feeding

PROMOTION OF BREAST FEEDING

- Antenatal advice
- Put baby to breast soon after delivery
- Demand feeds up to 3 hourly in first days
- Comfortable position for mother and baby
- Ensure good 'attachment'
- Professional and family support and encouragement
- Persuade stars of soap operas to breast feed on television

Infant feeding practices are dictated by fashion. Mothers may feel that breast feeding limits their social activities, spoils their clothes or is too difficult. Rich families in past ages employed wet nurses (e.g. Exodus 2; vii): today the bottle is more readily available. Around 60% of mothers breast feed after delivery, but this falls off in the first weeks. Seldom is there true failure of lactation. Women respond to information, advice and encouragement (Fig. 8.1). Nobody wants to see unwilling mothers browbeaten into breast feeding, but there is a happy medium between that and the indifference shown by many doctors and nurses.

Breast milk is nutritionally ideal for the term infant (Table 8.1). It is inexpensive, readily available, and convenient. Breast feeding, even for a month, gives an infant an excellent start to life. Protection from infection is important for survival in developing countries.

ANTI-INFECTION PROPERTIES OF BREAST MILK

- Sterile feed
- Maternal antibody (IgA)
- Lactoferrin
- Lysozyme
- Interferon
- Promotes colonization with lactobacilli and bifidobacter

Breast-fed babies may be fed *by the clock* (usually every 4 h). While lactation is established most recommend frequent *demand feeding*: after a feed the infant is allowed to rest, and the next feed is given when the infant wakes and appears hungry. Crying does not necessarily mean hunger: sleep does

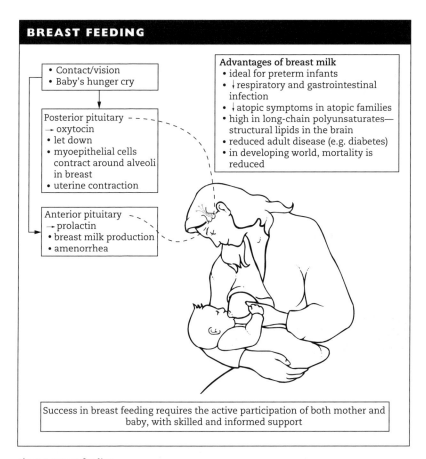

BREAST FEEDING

- Contact/vision
- Baby's hunger cry

Posterior pituitary
→ oxytocin
- let down
- myoepithelial cells contract around alveoli in breast
- uterine contraction

Anterior pituitary
→ prolactin
- breast milk production
- amenorrhea

Advantages of breast milk
- ideal for preterm infants
- ↓ respiratory and gastrointestinal infection
- ↓ atopic symptoms in atopic families
- high in long-chain polyunsaturates— structural lipids in the brain
- reduced adult disease (e.g. diabetes)
- in developing world, mortality is reduced

Success in breast feeding requires the active participation of both mother and baby, with skilled and informed support

Fig. 8.1 Breast feeding.

not necessarily mean satiation. Breast feeding can be a highly satisfying experience for the mother and infant. In the UK 60–70% of all mothers begin to breast feed, but only 40% of all mothers are feeding at 6 weeks, and only 25% at 3 months. Variation in rates is large: almost 90% of social class I mothers choose breast feeding. In the UK, breast feeding usually stops at 4–9 months, in the developing world, 2 years is the rule. There is, however, no evidence to suggest that bottle-fed babies are either nutritionally or emotionally deprived.

Many drugs are excreted in breast milk but maternal medication is only exceptionally a contraindication to breast feeding.

The *British National Formulary* offers advice on most drugs. Breast feeding is contraindicated with high-dose steroids, cytotoxic and immunosuppressive agents. Breast milk contains very little vitamin K (p. 57). Viral transmission means that breast feeding is contraindicated in known maternal HIV infection. 'Breast milk jaundice' is not a reason to stop (p. 71).

Formula feeds are available in two forms: whey dominant (60% whey) and casein dominant (30% whey). The former is more akin to breast milk and should be first choice. Each of the four UK milk manufacturers makes two milks so that a mother can change milks without changing company. There are no validated advantages to different manufacturer's milks, and parents should be dissuaded from constantly changing milk. Attention to detail in making up the feed is essential. Extra scoops, heaped scoops, packed scoops or additional cereal should be avoided. They add calories which encourage obesity, and extra solutes which cause thirst and irritability. It is conventional to warm feeds to approximately body temperature, but many babies will accept feeds direct from the refrigerator and come to no harm.

BOTTLE FEEDING REQUIREMENTS

• Meticulous care in hygiene

• Sterilizing bottles

• Correct feed reconstitution (e.g. 4-oz bottle).
  ◆ Take 4 oz cooled boiled tap water
  ◆ Fill scoop without compressing powder
  ◆ Scrape scoop level with clean knife
  ◆ Add four scoops of powder
  ◆ Dissolve, allow to cool to about 37°C
  ◆ May be refrigerated
  ◆ Only rewarm once

---

[i]   Soya-based formulae now exceed 5% of the formula market. There is no evidence that their use prevents food allergy or atopic disease.

Feeds should be given either 4-hourly or on demand. The newborn baby will require feeding round the clock, but within a few weeks will drop the night feed. As long as a night feed is demanded, it must be given. Leaving him to cry is pointless and unkind.

Mixed feeding

The term *weaning* is variously used to mean taking the baby off the breast or introducing solid foods. The age at which foods other than milk are introduced has been influenced to some extent by fashion. A full-term baby receiving milk will not develop any nutritional deficiency within 4 months of birth but the majority of infants receive solids from 3 months onwards. Solids before 3 months are ill advised. Recommendations are that mixed feeding should be achieved between 4 and 6 months.

• Use pureed fruit, vegetable and cereals as first foods.

• Ensure an adequate introduction of food containing protein and iron.

• Introduce one new food at a time, starting with small quantities.

• If a new food is not accepted by the infant, try something else. Feeding difficulties may stem from misguided insistence on food that she does not enjoy.

• Increase solid component of diet as chewing begins at around 6 months.

• The average 1-year-old will be having three main meals a day, with a small drink or snack mid-morning, mid-afternoon and at bedtime. Milk intake 20–30 oz/day.

Many mothers (and doctors) still use ounces:
1 fluid ounce = 28 mL
1 pint = 560 mL

Iron and vitamin supplements

Clinical vitamin deficiency states are rare and the healthy infant who receives adequate milk, and a mixed diet from 6 months, needs no vitamin supplements.

Folic acid is provided by leaf vegetables and fruits. Vitamin D may be derived from cholesterol through the action of sunlight. It is contained in oily (non-white) fish, liver and margarines. An increasing proportion of vitamin intake comes from 'fortified' foods: formula milk, bread, breakfast cereals, and fruit flavoured drinks. If parents choose to give a multivitamin supplement, it will do no harm. In prematurity, chronic illness, or poor diet, vitamin supplements are important.

Follow-on formula milk is available for infants from 6 months. They contain increased protein, calcium, and have added vitamins and iron.

> ℹ️ Iron deficiency anaemia occurs in around 15–25% of toddlers in areas of socioeconomic deprivation. It can be prevented with use of iron-enriched formula.

Nutrition of toddlers and schoolchildren

Changing social patterns in industrialized countries have had profound influences, not necessarily beneficial, on the nutrition of children. A tradition of home cooking, and indeed home growing of vegetables, has given place to supermarket shopping, fast and convenience foods and takeaway meals. Even in times and places of high unemployment this tends to persist. Increasingly, both parents seek work outside the home, and many families buy food that needs little more than heating up.

> Government policy:
> To reduce the average percentage of energy derived from fat to less than 35% by 2005.

Recent concerns about food additives — artificial flavourings, colourings, sweeteners, preservatives — and food allergies have turned some families towards 'natural' food and a return to home cooking.

The chief nutritional requirements of children are protein for building new tissue as they grow, and sufficient fat and carbohydrate to meet their substantial energy needs. Protein requirements (milk, egg, fish, meat, cereals and pulses) are about 1–1.5 g/kg/day. Energy requirements are high compared with most adults, who need less than a third of a child's requirements.

The dietary basis of obesity, dental caries and much constipation in childhood is well accepted. Refined sugar should be eaten in moderation, and sticky sweets preferably not at all (or at least not continuously!). An excess of fried foods (e.g. hamburgers and french fries) encourages obesity. Fibre helps prevent constipation. Most fizzy drinks ('pop'), so loved by children, have little or no nutritional value and help to rot teeth. Milk is highly nutritious (400 kcal/pint) but an excessive intake can contribute to obesity.

Energy requirements (kcal/kg/day)	
Maintenance	80
Growth	5
Physical activity	25
Total	110

Feeding problems

Early problems

Difficulties with feeding are common. In very young infants they may be to do with bottles, but at all ages they are more often to do with battles. Feeding mismanagement in early life may present with vomiting, disturbed bowel habit, unsatisfactory weight gain or crying. Most difficulties arise from one or more of three faults:

I The *quantity* of food is wrong. Both underfeeding and overfeeding may lead to vomiting and crying. In the first, weight gain is consistently poor. An overfed baby gains weight excessively to begin with, but may later lose. Overfeeding is more common in bottle-fed babies, partly because they are often fed to the limit of their capacity, partly because food has a sedative effect, and partly because of the mistaken belief that the biggest babies are the best.

2 The *kind* of food is wrong. Excessively early mixed feeding may lead to vomiting, diarrhoea and crying. A return to a milk diet will allow recovery, followed by cautious reintroduction of solids. Changing from one milk to another rarely achieves anything.

3 The feeding *technique* is wrong. Breast feeding requires expert help and advice. Difficulties with bottle feeding can only be recognized by watching the baby feeding. The baby may not be held comfortably: the bottle may be held at the wrong angle: the hole in the teat may be too small or too big: the milk may have been wrongly prepared. Instruction and advice provide the remedy.

Always check growth
You can quickly estimate expected weight:
Birthweight is regained after 10 days (1.5 weeks), thereafter babies gain 200 g/week for the first 3–4 months, e.g. 6 week old, birthweight 3.2 kg: 6 minus 1.5 = weeks spent growing $\Rightarrow$ 4.5 weeks at 200 g/week $\Rightarrow$ 900 g weight gain $\Rightarrow$ expected weight 3.2 kg + 0.9 kg = 4.1 kg

---

Infantile colic

Infantile colic, or evening colic, is a common problem arising in early life and lasting, as a rule, not beyond the age of 4 months. An otherwise placid baby devotes one part of the day, most commonly between the 6 pm and 10 pm feeds, to incessant crying. He may stop when picked up, but certainly cries again if put down. Attention to feeds, warmth, wet nappies, etc. is unavailing. The cause is unknown. First reassure and monitor growth. Anti-bubbling agents (Infacol) may be helpful. In extreme cases, some infants respond to a cow's-milk-free diet with a hydrolysed formula feed.

Sucking and feeding

Most babies take a feed in 20–30 min, but some drain their bottle in 5–10 min and may

then have filled their stomachs. Infants may find comfort in non-nutritive sucking on a thumb or a dummy. The widespread use of comforters (dummies) in the face of sometimes vehement opposition from the medical and nursing professions suggests that mothers have known this for a long time. The only hazard of dummies is as a vehicle for infection: they do not make teeth protrude.

From 6 months, an increasing diversity of foods and textures should be tried, and the child allowed to learn the joy of eating—even if this is not the tidiest of processes. Major conflict is best avoided. There is a delicate distinction between encouraging the conservative child to try something new, and coercing the reluctant child to eat 'what is good for him'. The mother who sits by the high chair supplying endless diversions whilst she subtly spoons in 'one for Sarah, one for Teddy', is more likely to be storing up trouble than solving a problem. The management of such problems lies in the patient, repeated but firm explanation to the parent that no normal child with access to food will starve: that children of some ages are dominated by the need for food, but at other ages it may be a low priority: that wise parents do not start battles with their children that they are bound to lose; and that a mother will often achieve most by doing least.

Obesity

Obesity in childhood is a common and troublesome problem—troublesome to the child, the family and the doctor. Some heavy-weight newborns seem to have insatiable appetites: their price for peace is food, and they seem doomed to obesity from the womb. In others, the tendency to excessive weight gain may appear in infancy, toddlerhood or during school years. Although only 10–20% of obese infants are still fat when they start school, half of all fat schoolchildren were overweight as babies and obesity may persist into adulthood. Fat children often come from fat families. Many fat children are gluttons, tucking away excessive calories, predominantly from carbohydrates. Equally, some fat children do not eat excessively. Similarly, some fat children take a lot of exercise, others none. Obese children are nearly always tall for their age. Obesity combined with short stature suggests an underlying pathology.

> Government policy:
> To reduce the prevalence of obesity in men to under 6% and in women to under 8% (adult obesity = body mass index > 30 kg/m²).

Obesity may limit exercise tolerance. In boys the disappearance of the penis into a pad of suprapubic fat may lead to a mistaken diagnosis of hypogonadism. The dominant symptoms are psychological. The fat child may be teased and ostracised, and the fat girl cannot buy fashionable clothes.

In obese children, weight reduction is advisable but impossible to procure without the enthusiastic collaboration of the child and their family. A limited-calorie diet, encouragement to exercise, and ample moral support form the basis of treatment. No specific foods should be forbidden, but the second slice of buttered toast must be eschewed. Group activities may help. Drugs are best avoided. Any emotional stresses at home or at school should if possible be alleviated. If satisfactory weight loss is achieved, follow-up should not be too short.

Defective nutrition

Nutritional deficiency may consist of a general shortage of food or a lack of specific dietary factors. Starvation is only seen in

Europe in children who have been grossly neglected, but in many parts of the world, especially the tropics and subtropics, *infantile marasmus* is all too common. In these areas, breast feeding is customarily continued for about 2 years, and there is very little alternative. If the supply of breast milk is inadequate, starvation ensues. The infant with marasmus is a prey to intercurrent infection, and mortality is high. There is also evidence that starvation in the first year of life, even if subsequently corrected, may cause permanent mental handicap.

Kwashiorkor, or protein dominant malnutrition, is seen in the same parts of the world as marasmus but in older children, usually 2–4-year-old. At this age the next baby often displaces the older sibling from the breast, and milk is replaced by a low protein starch- (rice or maize) based diet. The child is listless, the face, limbs and abdomen swell, the hair is sparse, dry and depigmented, and there are areas of hyperpigmentation ('black enamel paint') especially on the legs. Diarrhoea is sometimes a feature. Worldwide, vitamin deficiencies remain an appalling problem for children.

An increasing number of Western families are adopting bizarre diets in the name of religion or conservation. Growing children fed on such diets may be malnourished. That contrasts with the vegetarian diet: children in vegetarian families are healthy (and most unlikely to be obese).

> **i** Vitamin A deficiency is the single most important cause of childhood blindness worldwide. An estimated 250 000 young children each year suffer from xerophthalmia and nearly 10 million suffer from lesser degrees of deficiency. Supplementation is cheap, protective and reduces infection.

Rickets
Nutritional rickets results from dietary defi-

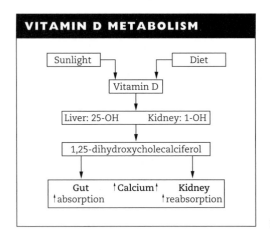

Fig. 8.2 Vitamin D metabolism.

ciency of vitamin D coupled with inadequate exposure to sunlight (Fig. 8.2). It presents at times of active growth—in the pre-school years of life and at puberty. It is more common in Muslim children in the UK because the traditional diet is poor in calcium and they receive little sunlight on their skin.

Deficiency of calcium, phosphorus or vitamin D interferes with bone maturation beyond the stage of provisional calcification which therefore tends to accumulate as osteoid tissue, especially at the epiphyses where active growth is most rapid. This accounts for the thickening of epiphyses seen particularly at the wrists, ankles and costochondral junctions ('rickety rosary'). The frontal bones may also be thickened. Toddlers develop bow legs: older children become knock-kneed. There is hypotonia. In malabsorption states rickets tends to develop after the diagnosis is made and growth is established because it is a disease of growing bones.

Serum calcium is normal or reduced and the alkaline phosphatase is raised. X-rays show broadening, cupping and rarefaction of the bone ends (Fig. 8.3).

Prevention of nutritional rickets can be assured by a daily vitamin D intake of 400 i.u. All baby milk foods and most cereals have vitamin D added. Treatment of established cases requires education regarding the diet, and supplementary vitamin D.

Renal Rickets has two main origins:
• *Glomerular* disease in chronic renal failure leads to failure of hydroxylation in the kidney to the active 1,25-dihydroxycholecalciferol.
• *Tubular* renal rickets. Failure of normal tubular reabsorption of phosphate occurs (e.g. vitamin D-resistant rickets).

Scurvy

Scurvy is now a very rare disease. It is also rare in countries where fruit is plentiful. The predominant symptom of scurvy is haemorrhage, into the gums, the skin or subperiosteally. X-rays show periosteal elevation and, later, calcification of subperiosteal haemorrhages. There is a rapid response to vitamin C.

RICKETS

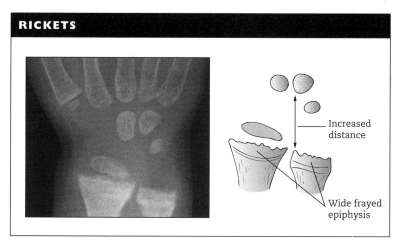

Fig. 8.3 X-ray of wrist showing rickets.

NUTRITIONAL ASPECTS OF CHRONIC DISEASE

Condition	Problems	Management
Severe cerebral palsy	Poor oromotor skills Gastro-oesophageal reflux Constipation Rejection by family	Protein/kCal supplements Avoid obesity Treat reflux/constipation Nasogastric/gastrostomy feeding Family support

Cystic fibrosis	Protein fat malabsorption
	Recurrent infection
	High energy demands
	Loss of appetite
		High energy intake (150% of
		    average needs for age)
		Do not use a low fat diet
		Pancreatic enzymes
		Fat soluble vitamins
		Aggressive management of
		    infection

Chronic renal failure	Anorexia/ill-health
	Renal osteodystrophy
	Poor vitamin D
	    hydroxylation
	Poor phosphate excretion
	Low calcium
	Hyperparathyroidism
		Energy supplements
		Nasogastric/gastrostomy
		    feeding
		Controlled protein intake
		Phosphate restriction
		Vitamin D and Ca

Childhood malignancy	Anorexia Recurrent ill-health Vomiting	Protein/energy supplements Intensive nutritional support Anti-emetics

Table 8.2 Nutritional aspects of some childhood conditions.

Nutrition in chronic disease

In many chronic diseases of childhood, nutritional care is an essential part of management (Table 8.2). Careful monitoring of growth is mandatory. The paediatrician should be a source of support, information, and advice for the family. A multi-disciplinary approach is needed—do not meddle with a young child's diet without dietetic help!

OSCE Station: History taking—feeding

Clinical approach:

- begin with open questions (e.g. could you tell me what worries you?)
- then focus to more specific questions

Diet
- breast/bottle feed
- mix or milk and solids
- quantity and frequency
- any specific exclusions
- nutritional supplements
  ◇ vitamins
  ◇ specially modified milk

Feeding
- bottled milk made appropriately
- who feeds him/her
- time taken to feed
- enjoys meal times
- appropriate for age

Appetite
- keen and hungry, wants more
- comparison with other children

Associated symptoms:
- weight gain
- tiredness, lethargy
- abdominal pain
- vomiting
- diarrhoea/constipation

Kelly-Marie is 5 months old. Her mother is very concerned because she is not feeding. Please take a short history

- the main concern: she is not getting any food into her
- normal birthweight and neonatal history
- artificial formula feeds: 6–8oz, 3–4 hourly
- solids at $2^{1}/_{2}$ months
- 'not feeding at all'
- 'vomits most feeds'
- stool: 3/day
- stool a little loose
- generally happy
- first child
- single mother

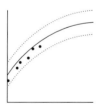

- normal growth
- normal development

It is likely that these symptoms relate to the way Kelly-Marie is being fed. The feeding problem, with normal growth, does not suggest underlying disease

Never forget:

- say hello and introduce yourself
- tell the parent(s) and child what you aim to do
- general health—is the child ill?
- ask, is there anything else you think I should know?

If asked or time permits:

- full history
- do not forget:
  ◇ birth history
  ◇ development
  ◇ immunizations
  ◇ family/social
  ◇ history

Look around for:

- general evidence of care or neglect
- dietary supplements
- growth charts; has mother got the child health record (red book)?

Special points

- diet is what you eat, appetite is whether you eat it
- if you wish, make notes
- current recommendations are for introduction of solids at 4 months, but almost everyone gives some solids at 3 months
- the mother is usually a member of staff who has been given a history

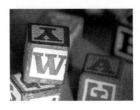

Abnormal Growth and Sex Development

Abnormal growth

Failure to thrive

> ## CAUSES OF FAILURE TO THRIVE
>
> - Inadequate food intake:
>   - Feeding problems or neglect
>   - Poor appetite
>   - Mechanical problems, e.g. cleft palate, cerebral palsy
>
> - Vomiting
>   - Gastro-oesophageal reflux, pyloric stenosis
>   - Feeding problems
>   - Food intolerance
>
> - Defects of digestion or absorption
>   - Cystic fibrosis
>   - Food intolerance (including coeliac disease)
>   - Chronic infective diarrhoea
>
> - Failure of utilization
>   - Chronic infections
>   - Heart failure, renal failure
>   - Metabolic disorder
>
> - Emotional deprivation

The term is applied to a child in the first year or two of life whose predominant symptom is unsatisfactory weight gain and growth (Fig. 9.1). Careful history and examination is essential. Initial investigations include blood count, tests of renal and liver function, acute phase response (ESR, CRP or plasma viscosity), coeliac disease antibodies and, in girls, chromosomes.

Sometimes the main reason for failure to thrive is obvious—inadequate food intake or chronic vomiting or diarrhoea. A good history, physical examination and check of the urine are mandatory. Often there is no clear reason apparent at the first consultation: parents appear caring and competent, adequate food is given, and there is no dramatic story suggesting any particular disorder. Solving the problem is difficult and unfocused investigation is not helpful. The parent-held Child Health Record (the red book) gives invaluable information about growth. Community health workers (e.g. the health visitor) can provide a reliable account of the home and whether both food and emotional nourishment are available there. A home visit can be most revealing. It may be necessary to admit the child to hospital to be fed standard amounts of food and observed to see if weight gain occurs, and to note symptoms. At the same time basic screening tests can be performed on the blood and urine to exclude infection and other common disorders. If these tests are negative, and the child is still failing to thrive, tests for rarer disorders including the syndromes of malabsorption become necessary.

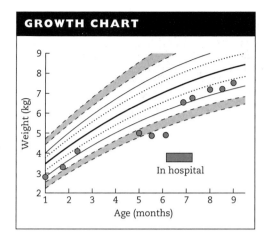

GROWTH CHART

Fig. 9.1 Sadie was admitted at 5 months of age with failure to thrive. In hospital she gained weight well with normal feeding and was discharged with intensive community based support.

Short stature

The majority of children presenting with short stature are normal, short children. Some of them were born small for gestational age and many have short relatives including one or both parents. In healthy short children, growth velocity is normal, as shown by serial measurements plotted on a centile chart. Growth velocity can be measured more accurately over 6–12 months and plotted on a growth velocity chart. The commonest reason for a child being short is having short parents. The child's height centile should be compared with their parents. Delayed puberty (often familial) with delayed bone age is common; the later pubertal growth spurt allows these children to catch up. Children with a height below the 2nd centile (2 SD below mean), or a reduced growth velocity require careful assessment. The single greatest challenge is to distinguish those with organic pathology from the many children with *non-organic failure to thrive*—an important group whose problems are social, emotional or economic in origin.

CALCULATE THE MID PARENTAL HEIGHT (MPH) AND TARGET CENTILE RANGE (TCR)

Example: A girl with short stature, mother 154 cm, father 170 cm.
• Reduce father's height by mean difference between male and female heights: 14 cm. Father (adjusted) = 156 cm.
• MPH = mean of mother and father (adjusted) = 155 cm.
• TCR = MPH ± 10 cm.
• Plot TCR + MPH on growth chart at 18 years.

For boys do the same but add 14 cm to mother's height.

Congenital hypothyroidism is detected by neonatal screening (p. 213), but acquired hypothyroidism in older children commonly presents with short stature. Growth hormone (GH) deficiency may be isolated or part of a wider pituitary insufficiency, and it may be complete or partial. Random GH levels are of little use. Diagnosis of GH deficiency requires complex tests. Bone age is retarded in both pituitary and thyroid deficiency, but especially in hypothyroidism.

CAUSES OF PATHOLOGICAL SHORT STATURE

- Defects of nutrition, digestion or absorption.
- Social and emotional deprivation.
- Most malformation syndromes.
- Chronic disease (e.g. renal insufficiency, malignancy).
- In girls, abnormalities of the X chromosome (Turner's).
- Deficiency of thyroid or growth hormone.
- Long-term steroid therapy.
- Disorders of bone growth (e.g. skeletal dysplasias).

Catch-up growth is seen in young children in whom the cause of retarded growth has been removed or corrected (Fig. 9.2). Growth accelerates as the appropriate growth centile is reached. In infants and young children, catch-up growth can be complete: thus a 4-year-old whose growth has been suppressed by high doses of prednisolone will regain normal height once the steroid therapy is decreased or stopped. However, as puberty nears catch-up growth may be incomplete so that permanent stunting may occur from temporary factors which have stunted growth.

ENDOCRINE INVESTIGATIONS IN SHORT STATURE

- Bone age
- Thyroid function tests
- Cortisol studies
- GH stimulation (e.g. glucagon/clonidine).

Tall stature

Children who are entering puberty early or who are overweight tend to be relatively tall (90–97th centile). Children with heights well above the 97th centile usually come

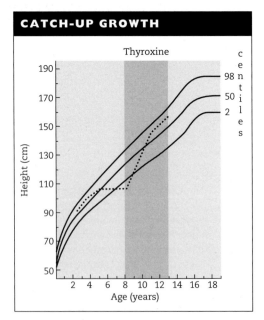

CATCH-UP GROWTH

Fig. 9.2 Catch-up growth. This boy developed hypothyroidism which was diagnosed at the age of 8. He showed excellent catch-up growth with replacement therapy.

from tall families. Formulae exist to calculate approximate final height from present height, age and bone age. If height is going to exceed socially acceptable limits, exceptionally hormone therapy is used to finish the growth process prematurely. This requires careful consideration of career and recreational aspirations (ballet or basketball?).

Rarer causes of tall stature include *Klinefelter's syndrome* (p. 90) and *Marfan's syndrome*. True Marfan's syndrome is an autosomal dominant disorder of connective tissue with slender habitus, arachnodactyly, typical facial appearance and a propensity to dislocated lenses, prolapsing mitral valve and dissecting aneurysm of the aorta. There are also 'marfanoid' families and individuals who are long and thin but not liable to complications.

Abnormal sex development

Intersex
The term is used to describe conditions in which the external genitalia at birth are not clearly male or female: some are masculinized genetic females; others are incompletely masculinized genetic males. The diagnostic problem is extremely urgent, partly because the most common underlying disorder is dangerous congenital adrenal hyperplasia (p. 213)—and partly because prolonged uncertainty about the true sex is intolerable for the parents. No-one should assign sex at birth if they are not sure, much harm may be done if the wrong sex is assigned: later reversal may be traumatic. The 'right' sex is determined more by anatomy (functional possibilities) than by genetics.

Intersex is rare. True *hermaphrodites* (with ovarian and testicular tissue) may have indeterminate genitalia. Investigation of intersex begins with karyotyping, ultrasonography and steroid chemistry.

Testicular feminization (androgen insensitivity) syndrome
Abnormalities at the androgen receptor result in genetic males with testicles, but the external genitalia of a female pattern. Inguinal herniae are typical and sometimes testes are palpable in the labia majora. At puberty normal female secondary sexual characteristics develop with amenorrhoea. Orchidectomy is advised later because of a risk of malignant change. The androgen receptor is on the X chromosome and there is a recurrence risk amongst siblings.

Turner's syndrome
Turner's syndrome occurs in 1 in 2500 girls (Fig. 9.3). The characteristic karyotype is 45XO (one X chromosome is lacking), but deletions or mosaicism involving the X chromosome may also be found. At birth the only noticeable abnormality may be lymphoedema of the legs. More character-

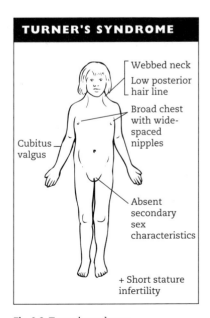

TURNER'S SYNDROME

Webbed neck
Low posterior hair line
Broad chest with wide-spaced nipples
Cubitus valgus
Absent secondary sex characteristics
+ Short stature infertility

Fig. 9.3 Turner's syndrome.

istic features may be apparent later. Coarctation of the aorta should be excluded. Secondary sexual characteristics rarely appear: the uterus and vagina may be small and the gonads by rudimentary streaks in the edge of the broad ligament. Breast development and menstrual periods may be induced by hormone therapy. Affected individuals remain infertile and short (few exceed 1.5 m or 5 feet) but in some girls growth hormone may improve stature. Intelligence is normal in most.

Klinefelter's syndrome

Characteristic karyotype is 47XXY, but mosaicism may be found. Although this condition occurs in 1 in 500 males, most are not detected until late childhood or adult life. The small testicles, long limbs and female habitus are rarely noticed early in life. Spermatogenesis is always impaired and infertility is usual.

Late and early puberty

Girls reach puberty on average a year before boys (p. 29). The age of puberty is influenced by genetic and environmental factors (Table 9.1).

Children (especially boys) and their parents frequently seek advice about 'late puberty'. The absence of any signs of puberty at the age of 14 in girls and 16 in boys does not necessarily require investigation especially if there is a family tendency to late puberty. The measurement of height is useful, for physiological delay is more probable in short boys. In short girls with delayed puberty, it is important to exclude Turner's syndrome. The vast majority of children with 'late' puberty are normal: they need

AGE OF PUBERTY		
	3rd centile	97th centile
Girls	8 years	13.4 years
Boys	9 years	13.8 years

Table 9.1 Age of puberty in UK.

reassurance, moral support and patience. Exceptionally, induction of puberty is indicated if there is pituitary or gonadal insufficiency.

Precocious puberty is the development of secondary sexual characteristics before 8 years in a girl or 9 years in a boy. True (central) precocious puberty results from premature secretion of gonadotrophins and follows the normal pattern of development. In gonadotrophin independent precocious puberty (e.g. congenital adrenal hyperplasia, adrenal tumours, gonadal tumours) the sequence of pubertal changes may be abnormal. Isolated precocious development of breasts (*thelarche*) is less rare and commonly resolves, followed later by normal puberty. Intracranial tumours, hydrocephalus, meningitis and encephalitis may lead to precocious puberty.

Gynaecomastia in adolescent boys is almost always physiological and self-limiting. This does not prevent it being a considerable social embarrassment.

> **i** True precocious puberty is more common in girls. In boys it is more likely to be due to underlying pathology (e.g. brain tumour).

OSCE Station: Assessment of growth and nutrition

Clinical approach:

Check face
- colour
- anaemia

Check general appearance:
- bright and alert/unwell
- any dysmorphic features

Inspection
- is the child thin or obese?
- is muscle bulk normal?
- is body shape normal (e.g. cushingoid features)?

Height and weight
- ideally plot both on chart
- do height and weight match?

Pubertal status
- it may be inappropriate to undress the child
- can any assessment be made on inspection?
  - body shape
  - breast development
  - voice change
- full pubertal staging requires examination of the genitalia and breasts

---

Sophie is 4 years old. Please measure her height

- measuring device fixed to vertical wall
- in contact with wall
  - head
  - shoulder
  - buttocks
  - heels
- support head
  - looking forward
  - external acoustic meatus level with lower border of eye socket

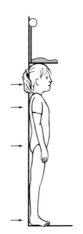

- feet flat on floor
- measuring device fixed to vertical wall
- you may be given a growth centile chart and asked to plot her height

Sophie may well be of normal height

Never forget:

- say hello and introduce yourself
- signs of chronic ill health
- mention the obvious (e.g. nasogastric tube, gastrostomy)

Look around for:

- growth and nutrition of parents or siblings
- is child clean and washed?
- has the child healthy hair and teeth?

Special points

- do not embarrass or upset the child or teenager (e.g. 'I notice that David is 16 years of age, very short, and has no signs of puberty')
- avoid terms like 'stunted'
- a good guide to obesity and thinness is inspection
- measure head circumference in all infants, and in children with neurological disease

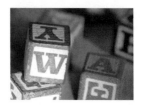

The Child with Learning Problems

A child's education is the equivalent of an adult's occupation, and is second only to the family in influencing a child's life. Children who get little support or encouragement at home may find more sympathy and understanding at school. It is therefore of great importance that:

• Children are in the best possible state of health — physical, mental and emotional — to benefit from their educational opportunities;

• Schools offer a sound basic curriculum with a wide variety of additional options in an environment which encourages learning and builds on success;

• Children leave school self-confident, healthy and with aspirations appropriate to their interests and to their educational achievements (which may not coincide with their parents' ambitions).

The educational system in the UK is a 'mixed economy' of state and private schools running side by side. The conventional pattern of education they offer will meet the needs of about four-fifths of all children. The remaining one-fifth, for a variety of reasons listed below, will need either some modification of the educational programme in mainstream schools or, if the problems are more severe, education in a special school designed, staffed and organized to meet their needs.

The main medical problems which can affect children's education may be considered in groups, and not infrequently children have problems in more than one group.

Physical — motor

Disorders such as cerebral palsy (p. 112), muscular dystrophy and severe congenital abnormalities, especially of the limbs. Children with restricted mobility may not be able to join in games and physical education or to climb stairs. They need extra time to negotiate long corridors and may need handrails. Wheelchair users cannot negotiate stairs and need wide toilets. Problems of manipulation may prevent the use of normal writing implements: special pens or a computer may be needed.

Physical — sensory

Impaired vision or hearing present obvious barriers to education. If they are severe, and especially if they are combined (the deaf/blind), special equipment and specially trained teachers are necessary.

Mental

Children with moderately impaired intelligence are usually best served by the provision of extra help in the classroom (usually non-teaching aides) in mainstream schools. More severe impairment needs the facilities and specially trained staff of a special school.

Emotional

Emotional problems often reflect social problems at home. A few children are diffi-cult to motivate, in sharp contrast to the normally insatiable appetite for information in young children. Others are hyperactive, aggressive, destructive or antisocial. Not only are they difficult to teach; they disrupt the classroom and make the teacher's task well-nigh impossible.

Communication

In addition to deafness on the receptive side and the dysarthria of some forms of cerebral palsy on the expressive side there are a variety of poorly understood disor-ders, including autism (p. 126) and dyslexia (p. 98) which cause severe difficulties. The detailed diagnosis of these problems, and the devising of a suitable educational pro-gramme, call for very special skills.

Chronic illness

Chronic illness can interfere with edu-cation in a number of ways. Intractable asthma may result in frequent absences from school with resultant poor academic progress. Epilepsy may place a few restric-tions on physical activities. Diabetes and coeliac disease may affect meals taken at school. Chronic juvenile arthritis may limit physical activities.

Learning disability (mental handicap)

Intelligence is difficult to define, but it has to do with understanding, reasoning and the association of ideas. It is not closely related to memory or creativity, nor has it much to do with sociability, which may be conspicuous by its absence in the super-intelligent.

Intelligence can be measured by a wide variety of 'intelligence tests', the results of which are often expressed as intelligence quotients (IQ). Quotients are calculated as the child's functioning age as a percentage of their chronological age. The concept of a global IQ which reveals all we need to know about a child's learning ability has been replaced by more detailed testing of the several components of intelligence. This provides a more comprehensive picture of the particular strengths and weaknesses of the individual child, and hence an indication of the particular kinds of help needed.

If global IQ is measured in an unselected population, the distribution curve is ap-proximately Gaussian, with a longer tail to the left (low IQ) than to the right. Most people with IQs between 2 and 3 SDs below the mean are part of the normal dis-tribution curve, and have parents of low IQ. Most children with IQ < 3.5 SD below mean have some organic cause for their mental handicap, congenital or acquired.

Developmental delay

One of the main reasons for recommend-ing that all young children should undergo regular developmental assessment (p. 42) is to detect significant delay as early as pos-sible. Another reason is to reassure parents who are unnecessarily anxious about their child. Learning disability is likely to present as delayed development, unless there are physical features (e.g. Down's syndrome, microcephaly) which permit early predic-tion of handicap. Although all children with learning disability are late developers, the reverse is not necessarily true. It is usual to express a child's achievement in a particular field or ability as appropriate to the average child of a particular age (e.g. head control is at the 3 month level). Faced with a child who is reported or found to be late smiling, sitting, walking or talking, a full paediatric history is essential. The following points need particular attention:

CAUSES OF LEARNING DISABILITY

- Congenital 75%
  - Chromosome abnormalities (30%), e.g. Down's syndrome.
  - Metabolic disease (under 5%), usually recessively inherited, e.g. galactosaemia, phenylketonuria.
  - Neurocutaneous syndromes (under 5%), often dominantly inherited, e.g. tuberous sclerosis, neurofibromatosis.
  - Other genetic causes, e.g. X-linked mental handicap and some cases of microcephaly
  - Idiopathic—the cause cannot be identified.

- Acquired 25%
  - Prenatal, e.g. alcohol, infections (rubella, CMV).
  - Perinatal, e.g. prematurity, haemorrhage, hypoxia, meningitis, septicaemia, hyperbilirubinaemia, hypoglycaemia.
  - Postnatal, e.g. trauma, infection.

- Was the baby very premature? Has she spent long periods in hospital? Has she had proper care at home?
- Is she delayed in all developmental areas or only in selected aspects? A child with learning disability will be retarded in all areas, although gross motor development may be better than social and language development. A child whose development is normal in any area is unlikely to have learning disability.
- Can a specific cause be found for a specific delay? If speech is delayed, is she deaf? If walking is delayed, does she have muscular dystrophy?
- A single assessment, especially if the child is having an 'off' day, may be an inadequate basis for decision-making. Although delay in recognizing, for example, deafness, is to be avoided, it is equally important not to express anxieties or initiate investigations prematurely. Re-examination, when progress can be assessed, is often helpful.
- Progressive (degenerative) brain disease is rare. It is important to establish if skills were achieved and later lost.

Differential diagnosis

There are three stages in the diagnosis of a 'late developer':

- Is the delay significant or does the child fall within the range of normal?
- What is the nature of the problem—learning disability, deafness, social deprivation?
- What is the cause? This may be relevant to treatment and useful for genetic counselling. Investigation will include biochemical screening of blood and urine for metabolic disorders, serological tests for prenatal infections, and neuroradiological studies.

Management

Some causes of learning disability are preventable. Genetic counselling may prevent recurrence of autosomal recessive disorders: rubella immunization should be universal: neonates are screened for phenylketonuria and hypothyroidism (p. 61) and, in some centres, for rarer metabolic disorders; improvements in perinatal and neonatal care should help.

For most children with severe disability there is no cure. With modern health care, life expectancy is often normal. These circumstances place great strains on their families. Handicapped children can take up all the time and energies of both parents, leading to physical exhaustion (especially as the children get older and heavier), neglect of siblings and the breakdown of marriages. The problems are multiplied in single parent families.

The principles of management are to help the child to develop to his full potential, however little this may be, and to offer all possible help and support to the family. Many children with learning disability have additional problems such as cerebral palsy, epilepsy or deafness. Full assessment is therefore essential before any treatment programme is drawn up. Although the health services have an important role, it is the social and educational services which have the chief responsibilities for helping children with learning disability. Many systems have been devised for encouraging maximal progress. Some are variations on traditional methods which have been properly assessed. Some, which unfortunately attract great media attention, play (to their considerable profit) on the eternal hope of parents that a cure may be found. Doctors must be understanding of parents who decide to try unorthodox methods, and must be prepared to help pick up the pieces if disappointment follows.

The main forms of family support are:
• home visits by an individual who can become a friend and offer a shoulder to cry on, but is at the same time well informed about practicalities
• provision of equipment for use at home, from incontinence pads to bath hoists, and adaptations to the home such as ramps for wheelchair access, or downstairs toilets
• respite care, whereby the handicapped child periodically goes to stay with a foster family or into residential care
• financial assistance, such as Disability Living Allowance or help from the Family Fund.

Down's syndrome

This affects approximately 1 in every 600 pregnancies: is less frequent for younger women and more frequent for those over 35 years. Most children with Down's syndrome have an extra chromosome 21 resulting from non-disjunction at the time of gamete formation. A few result from translocation or other abnormality involving chromosome 21. Parents who are translocation carriers are at substantial risk of having further affected children.

Prenatal diagnosis is possible by culturing fetal cells obtained by amniocentesis or chorion villus sampling. Usually these tests are offered only to older couples and are not always taken up, so have made little impression on the birth prevalence of the condition. Non-invasive tests involving biochemical parameters (including *low* maternal serum AFP) and ultrasound scanning of the skin folds on the neck indicate those most at risk.

Although none of the characteristic features of Down's syndrome is pathognomonic, and any may be present in a normal child, the association of several features usually enables a clinical diagnosis to be made (Fig. 10.1). Recognition in very small preterm babies is more difficult, and the

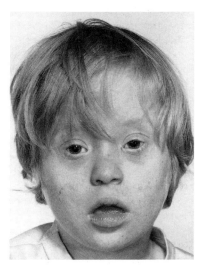

Fig. 10.1 A child with Down's syndrome.

condition is easily overlooked in aborted fetuses:

• The skull is brachycephalic; both face and occiput are flattened. At birth a 3rd fontanelle may be present, just anterior to the posterior fontanelle.

• Hypotonicity and hyperextensibility. All neonates with Down's syndrome are floppy.

• The palpebral fissures are slightly oblique with prominent epicanthic folds (hence the old term *mongol*). Tiny pale spots (*Brushfield spots*) appear on the iris as it becomes pigmented, forming a concentric ring around the pupil. The eyelashes are sparse. Squint, cataract and nystagmus are common.

• The mouth is small and drooping. After infancy the tongue becomes large and furrowed and often protrudes. The pinna may be an abnormal shape.

• The neck is short and broad with excess skin posteriorly.

• The hands and fingers are short. A single transverse palmar crease (*simian crease*) is common, as is a short, incurved little finger (*clinodactyly*). There is often a wide gap between the first and second toes, with a longitudinal plantar crease running from that gap.

• Short stature.

• Development is delayed in all aspects.

• Associated congenital abnormalities are common, particularly congenital heart disease (especially VSD and AV canal) and duodenal atresia or stenosis.

Diagnosis

This can usually be made with confidence on clinical grounds but should be confirmed by chromosome analysis, which is also necessary for genetic counselling.

Progress

Apart from any problems arising from associated congenital abnormalities, Down's babies may be difficult to feed in the early weeks. Thereafter they tend to be placid

and to thrive, although they have an excess of respiratory tract infections. Most are severely retarded and require special educational help. As adults they require continuing supervision. Their life expectancy is somewhat shorter than normal because they develop the degenerative disorders of advancing age a decade or two earlier than usual. Libido is diminished. No Down's male is known to have fathered a child: a few Down's females have borne children (half of whom, as expected, had Down's syndrome).

X-linked disability

More men than women are affected by non-specific learning disability, and in some families only males are affected. Several different forms of X-linked retardation are known, some of which are associated with macro orchidism. In one, a fragile site can be identified on the X chromosome, in which case it may be possible to identify female carriers or to diagnose affected males prenatally.

> **i**   *Fragile X syndrome* is the second commonest genetic cause of severe learning disability; Down's syndrome is the commonest.

Microcephaly

Primary microcephaly is associated with an inadequately developed brain at birth. The head circumference is small and increases abnormally slowly. The fontanelles close early. In severe cases, the infant has a characteristic appearance: the face is normal but the skull vault is disproportionately small. Some cases are genetic (autosomal recessive). Others are caused by intrauterine infections (rubella, cytomegalovirus), toxins (alcohol) or (rarely) radiation. If the brain is damaged in the perinatal period, the poor head growth will only become evident later.

Microcephaly must not be confused with craniosynostosis (p. 115). This is a disorder of fusion of sutures which will only result in a small head if it is neglected.

Disorders of speech and language

Normal speech development is described on p. 47. Medical advice may be sought about children who are late in beginning to talk, or whose speech is thought to be abnormal. Most of these children are, in fact, normal. Some children have a sizeable vocabulary before their first birthday while others say little until 3 or 4-year-old. A lisp is a common phase of speech development. Many 3- and 4-year-olds trip over their words because their thoughts and questions tumble out of their minds more quickly than they can articulate them. The average 4 year old asks 26 questions an hour!

Nevertheless it is important not to overlook a significant cause of delayed or abnormal speech. Furthermore, it is often helpful to refer any child with a speech problem to a speech therapist so that parents can be advised how best to help. The wrong kind of parental intervention can make the problem worse.

If speech development is delayed:
• Is the child being spoken to? Speech is learned by imitation.
• Can the child hear? Deafness is an important cause of speech delay. Less commonly, the hearing mechanism is intact but the brain cannot interpret the sounds heard.
• Are other spheres of development delayed? If so, learning disability must be considered.
• Is there evidence of emotional/behavioural disorder? Late speech is usual in autism (p. 126).
There is a strong link between language delay and later educational difficulties. A child with delayed speech should therefore be assessed as early and as expertly as possible.

The main abnormalities of speech are disorders of fluency (stammer/stutter) and of articulation. *Stammering* is common in young children and is much more common in boys than in girls. It usually goes spontaneously especially if it is ignored. If it persists into school age it becomes a barrier to communication and a social embarrassment. Speech therapy is helpful.

Articulation disorders are common in young children. If they persist or are severe, the child may be unintelligible. Speech therapy is essential for assessment and treatment.
• Consonant substitution (e.g. 'Come' is pronounced 'Tum').
• Nasality, resulting from cleft palate or nasopharyngeal incompetence. This may need surgical correction
• True dysarthria, as in some kinds of cerebral palsy (p. 112).
• Faulty enunciation, e.g. orthodontic problems or a wayward tongue may play a part.

School difficulties

There are many reasons for poor performance at school:
• Social/cultural. Parents who do not cooperate with the school and who do not encourage school attendance and school work.
• Neurological/psychological. Though major learning disability will usually have been detected before school age other disabilities of hearing, vision, fine motor skills, perception, and learning may not.
• Chronic ill health (e.g. asthma). It is important to check that the illnesses do warrant school absence.
• School refusal (school phobia) by an emotionally disturbed child, or truancy by

older children whose parents are usually unaware of the school absence until notified by the teacher, social worker or police.

If a healthy child of normal intelligence and good vision and hearing has educational difficulties, an emotional problem will often be found. There may be unhappiness at home, or at school (from bullying or fear), or parental over-expectation or indifference. Conversely, emotional problems may be the result of learning problems. A report from the school is an important part of the assessment of the schoolchild. More detailed assessment of intelligence and abilities by an educational psychologist will provide recommendations for remedial help.

Reading backwardness
The child's reading ability is more than 2 years behind that which is expected for his chronological age. This is a common condition of boys and girls, particularly in those from social classes IV and V, and in children with an overt neurological disorder or a mild neurodevelopmental fault.

Specific reading retardation
The child's reading age is more than 2 years behind their mental age (as measured by IQ testing). They are much worse at reading, speech and language than at other skills, and are particularly recalcitrant to treatment. This is commoner in boys and occurs in all social classes. It is not associated with neurological abnormalities. Some of these children are said to suffer from 'dyslexia', but the term is falling out of favour because of early inaccurate descriptions of it.

Severe clumsiness is another important cause of school difficulties. Apart from difficulty with dressing or physical activities, some clumsy children may have great difficulty with writing and drawing. They may be considered wrongly to be stupid or lazy. Their incoordination may represent a mild

form of cerebral palsy. Whatever the cause, once the problem is recognized the children can be taught to overcome many of their difficulties.

Special educational needs
The normal educational provision of mainstream schools meets the needs of over 80% of children. The rest need something more or something different. In the past, some of these children were labelled according to the nature of their problem (e.g. mental handicap, physical handicap, deaf) and were placed in special schools bearing similar labels. The rest tended to flounder in the bottom layer of mainstream schools, often leaving without any educational qualifications.

More recent policy rests on three principles:
• the earliest possible recognition or anticipation of special educational problems
• the detailed assessment of the child's needs through psychological, medical, social, parental and other reports
• the integration of children with special problems into mainstream schools, unless their educational needs would be better met in the setting of a special school.

Statement of Special Education Needs
There is a statutory duty to inform the education authorities, at the earliest opportunity, of any child who may have special needs. Education for such children may start as early as 2 years and is particularly important for children with visual or hearing impairment, who need to establish good methods of communication with teachers and other children before formal education is possible. All children with special needs undergo a comprehensive assessment which results in a report ('Statement') which is discussed with the parents and then forwarded to the education authorities who have the responsibility for the child's educational provisions and

any further assessment. The process of assessment is sometimes referred to as *statementing*.

> Nearly 3% of children at mainstream secondary school have statements of special educational needs.

Visual impairment

Severe visual impairment is a terrible handicap at any age. When it is congenital, or even when its origin is in the pre-school years, it presents a serious threat to satisfactory development and education.

Local authorities keep a register of children with severe visual problems so that the families can be helped and suitable education planned. Experienced home advisers from either the local authority or the RNIB (Royal National Institute for the Blind—a charitable organization) visit the family to provide continuing advice and support. They provide practical advice, e.g. 'Wear noisy shoes and give a running commentary about all your household activities so that she can understand and learn about the things she hears, sometimes smells and feels, but never sees'. Severe visual impair-

ment requires formal education by methods not involving the use of sight; the specialist schools for the blind teach braille. For children with sufficient sight to use educational material involving large print and type, there are residential schools for the 'partially sighted'. Both types of school are few in number, and the child is almost certain to be resident in one some distance from home.

Squint (strabismus)

Nearly 1 in 15 children have a squint when they commence school (Fig. 10.2). The incidence is even greater in children with brain damage or learning disability. Paralytic squints, caused by paralysis of one of the external ocular muscles, are unusual in children.

Most squints in children are non-paralytic (concomitant). In non-paralytic squint, there is a normal range of external ocular movements, and a constant angle of squint between the two eyes in all directions of gaze. In latent squint, there is extraocular muscle imbalance but the eyes do not deviate most of the time. A latent squint is not visible on inspection, difficult to diagnose and usually causes no problems. Examination for a squint is a special technique

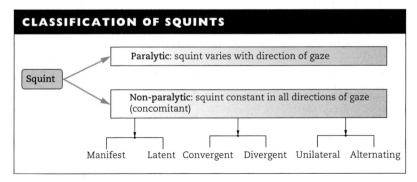

Fig. 10.2 Classification of squints. For example, one child may have a manifest, convergent, alternating non-paralytic squint.

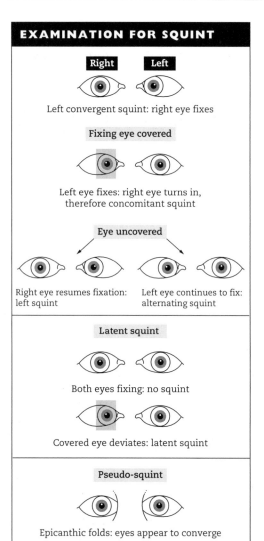

EXAMINATION FOR SQUINT

Right   Left

Left convergent squint: right eye fixes

Fixing eye covered

Left eye fixes: right eye turns in,
therefore concomitant squint

Eye uncovered

Right eye resumes fixation: Left eye continues to fix:
left squint   alternating squint

Latent squint

Both eyes fixing: no squint

Covered eye deviates: latent squint

Pseudo-squint

Epicanthic folds: eyes appear to converge

Fig. 10.3 Examination of the eyes for squint. The white dot on the pupil is the reflection of the examiner's torch.

and a favourite of undergraduate examinations (see OSCE, p. 102) (Fig. 10.3). Babies sometimes falsely give the impression of having a squint because of a low nasal bridge, epicanthic folds, or wide-spaced eyes (*hypertelorism*). This is a *pseudo squint* and is unimportant. A true squint which is manifest is always abnormal.

MOST SQUINTS ARE IDIOPATHIC

Rare causes include:
- Cataract
- Glaucoma
- Retinal disease
- Retinoblastoma

Any child with a squint should be referred to an eye specialist. Most importantly, a young child will suppress vision from the squinting eye in order to avoid blurred images and double vision. Unused, the eye can develop permanent *amblyopia* (diminished acuity of central vision). Treatment before school age should prevent this. If left untreated, vision will be lost in the squinting eye, denying the child binocular vision for life.

Refractive errors are common in children with squints. In many, early use of spectacles is sufficient treatment. Occlusion of the non-squinting eye is unpopular with children. The aim is to force the child to use the squinting eye. Patching or occlusion may be needed for several months. Severe squints may require surgery, if only for cosmetic reasons.

MANAGEMENT OF NON-PARALYTIC SQUINT

- Full ophthalmic examination
- Detection and correction of refractive error
- Patching or occlusion of the squinting eye
- Surgery

Hearing impairment

Hearing exists before birth and can be tested in neonates. They startle to a loud noise, or become quiet in response to a diminuendo growl. Neonatal screening with auditory evoked responses is proposed for universal neonatal screening. An infant's hearing is most easily tested at 7–8 months of age when the child has an insatiable curiosity for new sounds. All children should be tested at this age (p. 47). Appropriate tests are available for toddlers. Pure tone audiometry is not usually possible before 3–4 years.

Congenitally deaf babies babble normally

CAUSES OF DEAFNESS

- **Prenatal**
  - Maternal infection (rubella)
  - Malformation

- **Perinatal**
  - Hypoxia
  - Prematurity
  - Hyperbilirubinaemia

- **Postnatal**
  - Infection (meningitis, encephalitis)
  - Otitis
  - Ototoxic drugs

for about 6 months but then become quieter, do not talk but communicate by gesture. They may also have temper tantrums or other behavioural problems.

Most deaf children have some residual hearing, and so will be helped by a hearing aid which can be fitted as early as 3 months of age. That is the start of the treatment, not the end. The child requires prolonged exposure to speech and sounds at a level that she can hear with the hearing aid.

Skilled help is needed from a team of otologist, audiologist, hearing aid technician and specially trained teachers. Education for the deaf can be started from 2 years, but most deaf children will enter the partially hearing unit of a nursery school at 3–4 years and then progress to similar units attached to normal schools or to special schools for the deaf.

OSCE Station: Examination for squint

Clinical approach:

- check child understands you and is happy to cooperate
- note any obviously abnormal neurology

Inspection

- do eyes look healthy?
- symmetry
- normal facies

Acuity

- simple test that child can see with each eye (with glasses on if worn)
- does the child wear glasses?

External ocular movements

- child will follow light, toy or your face
- test in H pattern

Ophthalmoscopy

- red reflex
- are discs and retinae normal?—this can be very difficult, but attempt it

Light reflection

- hold light near your visual axis (on the end or your nose!)
- when child is fixing on light, is reflection in the middle of both pupils?

Cover test

- cover fixing eye
- squinting eye moves and fixes
- uncover the eye that was covered
- **Either** return to previous eye fixing **or** previously squinting eye fixes and other eye squints

---

Billy is 4 years old. Please examine him and tell me if he has a squint

He wears glasses

Acuity with glasses—identifies little pictures in book—normal

external ocular movements normal

R   L

asymmetric light reflection/ right eye fixes

left eye now fixes (right eye must be squinting)

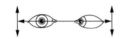

cover off: left eye returns to squinting + right eye fixes

Billy has a manifest, left, unilateral, convergent squint.

Never forget:

- say hello and introduce yourself
- general health
- quickly assess growth, nutrition and development
- mention the obvious (e.g. drip, leg in plaster)

Look around for:

- glasses
- eye patch
- eye drops

Special points

- pseudosquints are easily distinguished —the light reflection is symmetrical
- almost all squints are not due to ocular disease e.g. retinoblastoma
- latent squints are too difficult for medical students to find in an examination

Neurology

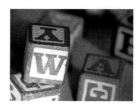

Brain growth and development occur early in life. Neurone formation is completed within 3 months of conception. Half the increase in head circumference between birth and adult life occurs in the first 18 months. Myelination is largely complete by the age of 3 years, and the establishment of dendritic connections by 5. The brain is particularly vulnerable in this early period.

Brain damage may be manifest as seizures (fits), cerebral palsy, learning disorders or behaviour problems. Progressive, degenerative brain disorders are rare. The spinal cord may be affected by congenital abnormality, infection or trauma. Peripheral neuropathy is extremely rare in children.

FACTORS AFFECTING BRAIN DEVELOPMENT

- **Genetic:**
  - ◆ Single gene defects (e.g. tuberous sclerosis)
  - ◆ Chromosome aberrations (e.g. Down's syndrome)

- **Prenatal:**
  - ◆ Drugs (e.g. alcohol)
  - ◆ Infections (e.g. rubella, HIV)

- **Perinatal:**
  - ◆ Extreme prematurity
  - ◆ Metabolic disturbances (e.g. hypoxia)

- **Postnatal:**
  - ◆ Infections (e.g. meningitis)
  - ◆ Trauma

Seizures

A seizure is the result of an abnormal paroxysmal discharge by cerebral neurones. The terms seizure, fit and convulsion are interchangeable. Fits are common in childhood: 6% of children have had a fit by the age of 11 years.

The pattern and prognosis varies with age.

Neonatal seizures
Seizures are common in the first month as a result of birth injury, metabolic and infective causes or developmental abnormalities (p. 74).

Infantile spasms
Infantile spasms are a rare and serious form of seizure characteristically commencing

SEIZURES

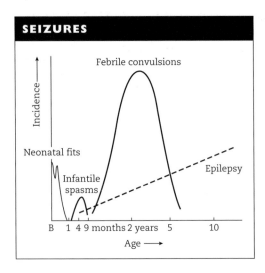

Fig. 11.1 The incidence and type of seizure at different ages.

between the ages of 1 month and 6 months (Fig. 11.1). The infant doubles up, flexing at the waist and neck, and flinging the arms forward—a *salaam spasm*; less commonly it is an extensor spasm. Associated mental handicap is common. The EEG usually shows a characteristically disorganized picture—*hypsarrhythmia*. Anticonvulsants or corticosteroids may suppress the fits. The final outcome is related to the cause, which may be metabolic or structural but often no cause is found.

Febrile convulsion

Febrile convulsion: a seizure occurring between 3 months and 5 years of age associated with fever but without evidence of intracranial infection or defined cause.

Four per cent of pre-school children have had a seizure; by far the commonest is a febrile convulsion. A family history of febrile seizures is often present.

They are precipitated by febrile illness and tend to occur at the start of the illness. Upper respiratory tract infections are the commonest association. The seizures are generalized with clonic movements usually lasting less than 10 min. The CNS is normal and there are no neurological signs once the seizure has ceased. One third will have further febrile convulsions with future illnesses, but very few have seizures after the age of 6. Prolonged, focal or frequent seizures, or an EEG which is abnormal more than 2 weeks after the seizure, suggest a diagnosis of epilepsy (recurrent *non-febrile* seizures).

Seizures are frightening to the family and it is common for the parents to think their child is dying. Therefore most dial 999 or rush their child to the local hospital.

Long-term management consists of explaining to the parents the relatively benign nature of febrile seizures and teaching them how to recognize and manage future seizures; how to use antipyretic agents safely and effectively; first aid for a seizure; and when and how to seek emergency assistance. Long-term prophylactic anticonvulsant therapy is occasionally used for selected children with recurrent febrile convulsions.

Idiopathic epilepsy

Recurrent non-febrile seizures of unknown cause.

MANAGEMENT OF A SEIZURE

- Recovery position: laying the child semiprone with the neck slightly extended so that secretions drain out of the mouth.
- If respiratory distress: open the airways by gently extending the neck, lifting the jaw forward. Do not put anything in the mouth. Give O_2 if available.
- If fit continues give diazepam: IV/IM/rectal.
- Check blood sugar
- Assessment and investigation. If there is any suspicion of meningitis, lumbar puncture is mandatory.

If the child is under 5 and febrile
- Cooling. Excess clothing or bedclothes should be removed. Occasional sponging with tepid water (which does not cause skin vasoconstriction) is needed. Paracetamol is helpful.
- Antibiotics, if an infection such as otitis media is present.

A seizure in a previously healthy child is usually associated with idiopathic epilepsy. About 1 in 200 schoolchildren are affected. The fits may be generalized or partial, and take a wide variety of forms: in between attacks the child is perfectly well. It is exceptional for the doctor to have an opportunity to witness a fit and the diagnosis rests principally on the history. Careful examination and appropriate investigation are essential; the EEG is consistently abnormal in 60%. Diagnosis can be difficult and it is important not to attach the label 'epileptic' to a child without good reason; it may be difficult to remove. It is very rare to identify serious brain disease or metabolic abnormality in a healthy child who has had a fit.

SEIZURE CLASSIFICATION

- Generalized
  - Tonic-clonic
  - Simple absences
  - Complex absences
  - Myoclonic

- Partial
  - Simple
  - Complex (consciousness ↓)
  - Partial + secondary generalized

Seizure classification

Generalized seizures

Tonic–clonic (Grand mal)
Major epileptic attacks classically comprise a tonic phase (continuous muscle spasm) which may start with a cry and, if prolonged, lead to cyanosis: then a clonic phase (jerking) which may be associated with tongue-biting and frothing at the mouth: then relaxation, unconsciousness and a period of drowsiness and/or confusion. Children often sleep after an attack. Indeed, any recurrent symptom or symptom-complex in a child which is regularly followed by sleep is likely to be an epileptic phenomenon. Most occur for no apparent reason. Flashing lights trigger fits in some children, usually when they are watching a malfunctioning TV screen or sitting very close to the TV. The EEG may show bilateral, slow-wave, subcortical seizure discharges. Major fits can last from less than a minute to over an hour (*status epilepticus*). Uncontrolled prolonged fits cause hypoxia, and may lead to brain damage, especially in the temporal lobes.

Status epilepticus occurs when a child fits continuously or repeatedly for over 30 min without recovering consciousness. Apart from external injury, hypoxic brain damage may result. Therefore all fits must be stopped fast; diazepam is the drug of choice. This is combined with securing an adequate airway, administering oxygen, protecting the child from injury and, over a longer period, maintaining fluid and electrolyte balance. At home, rectal diazepam or intramuscular paraldehyde are effective.

Absences

The onset of *simple absences* (*petit mal*) is always in childhood. It is not caused by organic brain damage and the intelligence and behaviour of the child are normal. An attack consists of a very brief absence of awareness lasting less than 5 s and accompanied by blinking. The eyes may roll up. The child does not fall down. He may present with school difficulties because of 'daydreaming' or inattention.

Absences may be provoked by encouraging the child to hyperventilate hard for 2 min. The characteristic EEG shows a 3 per second spike and wave pattern.

Complex absences tend to be longer, and associated with other movements and sensations. The prognosis is less good than for petit mal.

Myoclonic

The sudden brief jerks affect one part of the body, commonly arm or leg. They are a common feature in children who have other neurological disorders.

> The diagnosis of epilepsy is made on the history; listen to those who know the child.

Partial seizures

The seizure discharge starts in a focus of neurones. Sometimes the focus is at the site of previous cerebral damage (for example, as a result of anoxic damage to the temporal lobe during prolonged convulsions).

Simple

These occur without disturbance of consciousness. The convulsive movement predominantly affects one area only. Seizure activity may be focal and then 'march' up the affected limb and become more widespread (*Jacksonian seizure*). Sometimes the seizure is followed by temporary weakness of an involved limb (*Todd's paralysis*).

Complex (temporal lobe epilepsy)

Motor, sensory or emotional phenomena occur singly or in combination, together with impaired consciousness. The diagnosis is confirmed by EEG which commonly shows discharges from one temporal lobe.

General management of epilepsy

Although most seizures are idiopathic it is important to search for a primary cause from a careful history and examination, since seizures can be caused by space-occupying lesions, meningitis, hypoglycaemia, hypertension, and many other causes. A rare but interesting group are children with *neurocutaneous syndromes* in which a skin lesion is associated with an intracranial lesion. Many of these are genetically determined and associated with learning difficulties. It is important to examine the child's skin carefully for the pathognomonic skin lesion: *Sturge–Weber syndrome*: port wine stain (p. 181). *Neurofibromatosis*: café-au-lait spots. *Tuberous sclerosis*: depigmented *ash leaf* shaped macules on the trunk and, later on, papules over the nose and face (*adenoma sebaceum*). Learning difficulties are usual.

Prophylactic anticonvulsant therapy is given to children with recurrent seizures, usually until the child has been fit-free for at least 2 years. The lowest dose of the safest drug that suppresses fits is used. The prognosis is good for children who are otherwise healthy, have a normal EEG and respond promptly to preventive therapy:

PROPHYLACTIC ANTICONVULSANTS

- Drugs of first choice
  - Carbamezapine
  - Valproate

- Reserve drugs
  - Clonazepam (myoclonic)
  - Ethosuximide (absences)
  - Vigabatrin (partial, infantile spasms)
  - Lamotrigine (tonic–clonic)

EPISODIC EVENTS

Age 1–4	Reflex anoxic seizures (brief cardiac asystole from vagal inhibition—pain) Breath-holding attacks Masturbation
Age 4–8	Benign paroxysmal vertigo Night terrors
Age 9–16	Faints Migraine Habit spasms (tics) Behavioural disorders—hysteria

Table 11.1 Other episodic events.

less good for those with learning problems or cerebral palsy, with persistent seizure activity on EEG, and in whom a variety of drugs, alone or in combination, fail to give adequate control.

Most children with epilepsy attend normal school: only a tiny minority have such intractable epilepsy that special schooling is required. It is important that the teachers know how to recognize and deal with any seizure. Although the child should take part in most activities he may need extra supervision for swimming, and it may be wise to prevent him from doing activities such as fishing, rope or rock climbing and canoeing. Some doctors forbid cycling in traffic if the child has had a seizure in the previous 2 years, though seizures are uncommon during concentrated activity.

Conditions simulating epilepsy

Of those being treated for epilepsy, 20% do not have genuine epilepsy. Some parents imagine/perceive episodes, others present false stories. Many children have unusual periodic events as a result of other conditions (Table 11.1). A careful history, confirmed by more than one observer, should lead to accurate diagnosis (Table 11.2).

Nocturnal episodes may be especially difficult to interpret. Overnight or prolonged EEG recordings can be helpful. Similarly, 24-h ECG recordings may be diagnostic especially if the episodes are related to exercise. A parent's video recording is valuable (Table 11.2).

Meningitis

This is essentially a disease of childhood—80% of all cases occur in the first 5 years of life. The younger the child, the more difficult is diagnosis and hence the greater is the risk of residual brain damage. The importance of considering the *possibility* of meningitis in any sick child cannot be over-emphasized. In infants, a delay of only hours in diagnosis can make the difference between complete and incomplete recovery. If there is any doubt about the possibility of meningitis, a diagnostic lumbar puncture is mandatory.

In children past infancy, *meningism* the classic sign of meningeal irritation may be present. Neck stiffness—a reluctance to flex the neck—may be demonstrated by

FAINTS AND SEIZURES

	Seizure	Faint
Age	Any	8–15 years
Timing	Day or night	Day
Situation	Commonly during inactivity	Standing (school assembly, church)
Prodrome	Brief (twitching, hallucinations, automatisms)	Long (dizziness, sweats, nausea)
Duration	Variable	Under 5 min
Tonic–clonic movement	Common	Rare
Colour change	May be cyanosis	Pallor
Injury (e.g. tongue-biting)	Common	Rare
Incontinent of urine	Common	Rare
Epilogue	Drowsiness, confusion or headache	Quick full recovery
	Rarely partial paralysis	Never paralysis

Table 11.2 Features differentiating a seizure from a faint (syncope).

Early symptoms of meningitis are non-specific:

All Ages
Fever
Vomiting
Drowsiness
Seizures

Infant
Fretfulness
High pitched cry
Bulging fontanelle

Child
Headache
Photophobia
Neck stiffness

encouraging the child to look at his feet or kiss his knee. Head retraction is a sign of advanced meningitis. Kernig's sign is often present, but its absence does not exclude meningitis. (Meningism alone is not diagnostic of meningitis, sometimes it may be caused by otitis media, tonsillitis, cervical adenitis, arthritis of the cervical spine or pneumonia) (Table 11.3).

Investigation

Prompt lumbar puncture is imperative. If signs suggest raised intracranial pressure, lumbar puncture may not be possible. Gram stain and differential cell count provide the most useful immediate information. Usually it is possible to differentiate a viral meningitis (lymphocytic) from a bacterial meningitis (purulent) from the CSF examination provided the child has not received recent antibiotics (Table 11.4).

When the findings are equivocal it is usual to treat as if there is a bacterial pathogen. Faeces, CSF and throat swabs can be cultured for viruses, and in all cases blood culture should be performed. The rare, but serious tuberculous meningitis (p. 227) may present as a lymphocytic meningitis.

MENINGITIS		
1/3 Bacterial		**2/3 Viral**
Child	Newborn	All ages
Neisseria meningitidis (Gram –ve diplococcus) Strep pneumoniae (Gram +ve diplococcus) Haemophilus influenzae (Gram –ve coccobacillus)	Group B Streptoccus Listeria Escherichia coli Other coliforms	Enterovirus Adenovirus Epstein–Barr

Table 11.3 Causes of meningitis.

CHARACTERISTICS OF CSF			
	Normal	**Viral meningitis**	**Bacterial meningitis**
Appearance	Clear	Clear or hazy	Cloudy or purulent
Cells (mm^3)	0–4	20–1000	500–5000
Type	Lymphocytes	Lymphocytes	Neutrophils
Protein g/L	0.2–0.4	↑	↑↑
Glucose mmol/L	3–6	3–6	↓

Table 11.4 Characteristics of CSF in infants and children.

Treatment

Children with bacterial meningitis are treated initially with intravenous antibiotics. Until the bacterium has been identified cefotaxime is used. This is combined with supportive and symptomatic therapy—anticonvulsants, analgesics, or intravenous fluids for a collapsed child. Improvement should occur within 36h, and early treatment is usually associated with complete recovery though pneumococcal meningitis tends to follow a slower course. Viral meningitis is treated symptomatically.

Outcome

Bacterial meningitis is a serious condition: 5–10% of children die and 10% of survivors incur permanent brain damage resulting in deafness, cerebral palsy, hydrocephalus or epilepsy. Recurrent meningitis is most rare, and should provoke a close search for a dermal sinus: a small defect connecting the skin and the meninges. It is found in the midline on the head or down the back as far as the sacrum.

Viral meningitis has a much better prognosis; complete recovery is usual. Paralyses resulting from poliomyelitis, or deafness from mumps meningitis is hardly ever seen in countries that provide mass immunization.

Encephalitis

Encephalitis (inflammation of the brain) is associated with cerebral symptoms (e.g. fits and drowsiness) or neurological signs that are not accompanied by definite signs of meningitis (inflammation of the meninges). The CSF usually has raised protein and/or lymphocytes. The commonest form in childhood is acute disseminated encephalomyelitis (postinfectious encephalitis) usually occurring about a week after infection, e.g. chicken pox. Most cases are mild, but occasionally it is severe and brain damage results from demyelination. Encephalitis very rarely follows immunizing procedures (pertussis, measles); the risk is about 10 times smaller than that associated with the corresponding infection.

Herpes simplex encephalitis produces a wide variety of neurological symptoms. Electron microscopy of CSF, CT or MR scan and serology may be diagnostic. Acyclovir is given; intensive care may be needed. Over half the children acquire brain damage or die.

Chronic encephalitis may occur with HIV or following measles (*subacute sclerosing panencephalitis, SSPE*).

Acute post-infectious polyneuropathy

This is an uncommon condition which occurs shortly after acute infections. Over 2–4 weeks there is an ascending paralysis which progresses to a symmetrical peripheral neuritis with motor loss, sensory loss and absent tendon reflexes. If bulbar or respiratory muscles are involved, intensive care and ventilatory support is needed. Nearly all children recover fully, though this may take many months. The CSF is either normal or shows a high protein but normal cell count (*Guillain–Barré syndrome*).

Hydrocephalus

Hydrocephalus arises from obstruction of the normal CSF circulation either as a result of congenital abnormality, e.g. aqueduct stenosis or from postnatal causes such as meningitis, intracranial haemorrhage or tumour. Congenital neurological abnormalities are often associated with hydrocephalus (e.g. spina bifida).

In congenital hydrocephalus the size of the head at birth varies from normal to gross enlargement. As the CSF accumulates under pressure the head enlarges rapidly, the skull sutures separate, the anterior fontanelle bulges and the scalp veins appear prominent. The eyes turn downward (*setting sun sign*). In the older child whose skull sutures are united, obstruction to CSF pathways causes headache, vomiting and other symptoms of raised intracranial pressure. It is the *rate* of skull expansion rather than any single measurement that distinguishes the infant with hydrocephalus from the normal infant with a big head. The commonest cause of a big head is parents with big heads (Fig. 11.2).

Prompt surgical treatment is often needed. The usual practice is to bypass the obstruction by inserting a ventriculo-peritoneal shunt. Depending on the cause of the obstruction and the success of treatment, normal brain development and function is possible. Low grade infection and other technical problems often prevent the valves from being as permanently effective as desired (Fig. 11.3).

 Spina bifida has become rare due to:
- Improved nutrition
- Increased folic acid intake
- Prenatal diagnosis

Spina bifida

This congenital defect results from failure of closure of the posterior neuropore, which normally occurs around the 27th day of embryonic life.

The commonest and most severe form is a *meningomyelocele* (myelocele) in which elements of the spinal cord and nerve roots are involved. It may occur at any spinal level but the usual site is the lumbar region. The baby is born with a raw swelling over the spine in which the malformed spinal cord is either exposed or covered by a fragile membrane.

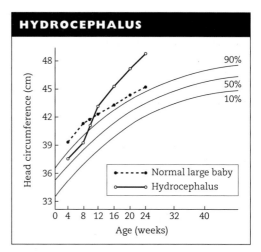

HYDROCEPHALUS

Fig. 11.2 The head circumference of a normal large baby increases at a rate parallel to the centile lines; in the child with hydrocephalus, head circumference increases at an abnormal rate.

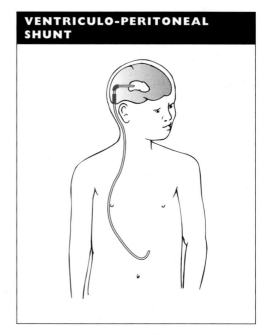

VENTRICULO-PERITONEAL SHUNT

Fig. 11.3 If hydrocephalus is progressive, CSF can be drained from the lateral ventricle to the peritoneal cavity. The ventriculo-peritoneal shunt is tunnelled under the skin, and can be felt behind the ear.

The majority are associated with hydrocephalus, particularly as a result of the *Arnold–Chiari malformation* in which a tongue, of malformed medulla and cerebellum, protrudes down through the foramen magnum, preventing free escape of CSF from the 4th ventricle.

The main physical problems from meningomyelocele are:
• Legs—paralysis below the level of the lesion, with associated sensory loss, hip dislocation and leg deformities (club foot).
• Head—hydrocephalus with learning problems.

• Bladder—neuropathic bladder with incontinence. Recurrent urinary tract infections may lead to kidney damage.
• Paralysis of the anus resulting in faecal incontinence.
The emotional and social problems for the child and family are massive, varying from the frequent hospital admissions and attendances to the problems of providing suitable education for a paraplegic, incontinent child.

Meningocele

This is less common and less serious. The sac of CSF is covered by meninges and skin and contains no neural tissue. Cosmetic surgery is not urgent.

Encephalocele

Encephaloceles are protrusions of brain through the skull, covered by skin, usually in the occipital region. If large, they are likely to be associated with severe brain abnormality.

Spina bifida occulta

Spinal X-rays of young children often show an apparent defect of the neural arches of the lower lumbar vertebrae, but there is usually a cartilaginous bridge which calcifies later. This is common and is not associated with signs or symptoms. True spina bifida occulta is sometimes associated with neurological problems; if there is an external 'marker' in the lumbar region (hairy tuft, naevus, lipoma), intraspinal pathology is more probable.

Cerebral palsy

A disorder of posture and movement resulting from a non-progressive lesion of the developing brain.

The term is rarely applied to brain lesions incurred after the age of 2 years. It occurs once in every 1500 live births.

The basic pathology may be a developmental abnormality, pre- or postnatal brain infection, physical or chemical injury to the brain, or a vascular accident (Fig. 11.4).

CAUSES OF CEREBRAL PALSY	
Prenatal	85%
Perinatal	10%
Postnatal	5%

The presentation varies according to severity. In the most severe cases poor sucking or altered muscle tone may arouse suspicion soon after birth. More often cerebral palsy is first suspected when the child's motor development is delayed—there may be poor head control or lateness in sitting. It is important to realize that, although the brain lesion is fixed and non-progressive, the disorder it causes varies in the early years as different movement patterns are acquired or persist beyond their time. A hypotonic infant may become hypertonic during the first year of life .

Terminology

• *Tone:* resistance to passive movement. Increased tone may be of two kinds, spasticity or rigidity.
  ♦ *Spasticity* arises from a lesion of the cortex or pyramidal tract pathways. The increase in tone is found in one direction only, e.g. supination of the forearm, not pronation; dorsiflexion of the wrist, not plantar flexion. Spasticity is often associated with increased reflexes and clonus. It is the commonest feature of cerebral palsy.
  ♦ *Rigidity* arises from a lesion of the basal ganglia or extrapyramidal pathways. The increase in tone is present in all direc-

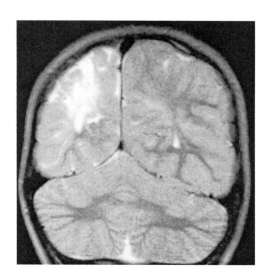

Fig. 11.4 This brain MRI shows an asymmetric lesion which led to a hemiplegic cerebral palsy.

tions and sometimes has a cogwheel feel to it.

• *Involuntary movements* (dyskinesia). These may be choreiform, athetoid or dystonic. The difference between them is sometimes quite subtle, the choreiform movements being of a more jerky nature than the sinuous athetoid movements. Dystonia tends to cause twisting movements involving part, or the whole, of the body.

• *Ataxia.* This manifests itself as a tremor on intention, difficulty in walking heel-to-toe, nystagmus and dysarthria.

Cerebral palsy may be defined by the distribution of the motor defect.

• *Diplegia.* Predominant involvement of the legs, though the arms may also be affected.

• *Quadriplegia.* Involvement of all four limbs.

• *Hemiplegia.* Involvement of one arm and one leg on the same side (Fig. 11.5).

Management

Early comprehensive assessment is essential because:

• There is often other associated handicap, e.g. learning difficulties, epilepsy, defects of vision and hearing;

• Disordered posture and movement can lead to permanent deformities;

• Cerebral palsy can present major problems of management at home and at school. Therefore apart from a detailed history and general examination the following have to be assessed: vision, hearing and intelligence, and the emotional and social state of the child and home. Usually the assessment and therapy are organized by the multidisciplinary team of the *Child Development Centre.* Early physiotherapy aims to establish a normal pattern of movement by facilitating normal postural reflexes and inhibiting the awkward persisting primitive reflexes, and to prevent deformity. Orthopaedic and neurosurgical intervention may be helpful.

Prognosis

This depends mainly on the presence or absence of associated handicaps, and in particular on the intelligence of the child. With normal intelligence, the problems of the most severe motor handicaps may be overcome. The quality of the management itself affects the prognosis. A severely affected child may require education in a special school where expert physiotherapy, occu-

ABNORMAL GAITS

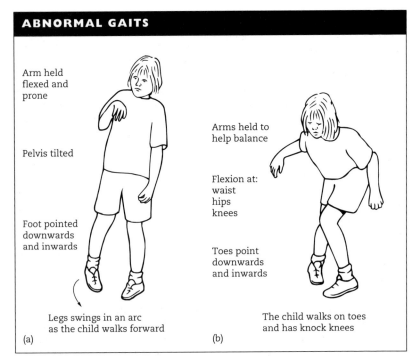

Arm held flexed and prone

Pelvis tilted

Foot pointed downwards and inwards

Legs swings in an arc as the child walks forward

(a)

Arms held to help balance

Flexion at:
waist
hips
knees

Toes point downwards and inwards

The child walks on toes and has knock knees

(b)

Fig.11.5 Abnormal gaits in children with (a) hemiplegia and (b) diplegia.

pational therapy, teaching and other facilities are available.

Children less severely affected, often those with hemiplegia, manage at normal school, and the least severely affected of all do not always reach the specialist. Their clumsiness, their inability to march in step or their difficulty in copying shapes may make them an object of derision at school without it being realized that they are suffering from mild cerebral palsy.

Space-occupying lesions

When symptoms occur they often follow raised intracranial pressure due to CSF drainage. Headache, misery and irritability are common early symptoms and are followed by unsteadiness, vomiting and visual disturbances. Fits may occur.

In infancy the anterior fontanelle is tense and the skull sutures widened. In older children, papilloedema occurs early. In any child suspected of having a space-occupying lesion, CT or MR brain imaging must be carried out promptly.

SPACE-OCCUPYING LESIONS

- Neoplasm

- Cerebral abscess
  - Otitis media
  - Meningitis
  - Infected emboli

- Subdural haematoma
  - Accidents
  - Non-accidental injury, shaking (p. 234)

Craniosynostosis (craniostenosis)

Premature fusion of one or more of the skull sutures results in an unusual-shaped head and may compress the brain or cranial nerves. The prognosis depends upon which sutures are affected. Premature fusion of all sutures results in a bulging forehead, proptosis and brain compression which requires urgent surgery. Premature fusion of a single suture, usually the sagittal, causes a misshapen head which may require surgery for cosmetic reasons. The cause is unknown. Sometimes there is a hereditary factor, and frequently there are associated skeletal abnormalities. The diagnosis is confirmed by skull X-ray or CT.

Plagiocephaly

Natural skull asymmetry is common in early infancy, but the sutures and fontanelles are normal; one side of the forehead and occiput are displaced forward. The asymmetry becomes less with growth and does not cause problems. There may be associated chest asymmetry.

Progressive neuromuscular disorders

Among the most distressing disorders of childhood are those that strike a previously healthy child and progress inexorably towards incapacity and death over months or, more often, years. They may affect principally the brain, the spinal cord or the muscles; many are genetically determined and few are open to effective treatment.

Progressive brain degeneration can result from several different conditions, many of which are due to autosomal recessive genes. They can be grouped into those that affect the grey matter (e.g. the *lipidoses* such as *Tay-Sachs disease*) and those that affect the white matter (*leucodystrophies*). They

present with loss of previously acquired skills, usually in the first two years of life; in general, the earlier the onset, the more rapid the progress.

Spinal muscular atrophies are a group of conditions due to autosomal recessive genes which present with progressive weakness affecting predominantly the lower half of the body. The infantile form of spinal muscular atrophy (*Werdnig–Hoffmann disease*) is evident from birth and progresses to death within a year or so; forms with later onset progress more slowly. Those with onset in late childhood often enjoy a reasonably active adult life.

Myopathies (muscular dystrophies) are also variable in their age of onset, rate of progress and mode of inheritance.

Duchenne muscular dystrophy

This is the commonest type of muscular dystrophy. It is due to an X-linked recessive gene and therefore only affects boys. The genetic abnormality is a deletion in the gene for dystrophin, a protein essential for muscle function. The condition presents as late walking (over 18 months), with an abnormal waddling gait or with difficulty climbing stairs. There is often marked lumbar lordosis. Affected boys develop enlargement of the calves due to fatty infiltration (*pseudo hypertrophy*) with absent knee jerks.

The ability to walk is lost about the age of 10 years and death occurs in early adulthood due to pneumonia or myocardial involvement. A proportion have intellectual impairment. A grossly elevated serum creatine phosphokinase level is present from birth.

In Duchenne dystrophy, boys asked to stand up from sitting on the floor, turn over onto all fours, and then 'climb up their legs'. This is *Gower's sign* (p. 38).

With the milder form of pseudohypertrophic muscular dystrophy (*Becker*) symptoms develop later and disability is mild.

There is no cure for muscular dystrophy. Therapy is supportive and there should be active physiotherapy and mechanical supports to prevent contractures and deformity and to maintain mobility for as long as possible. Obesity is to be avoided. Precise clinical and genetic diagnosis is important in order to provide reliable genetic counselling and allow antenatal diagnosis in future pregnancies.

Other progressive disorders

Rett syndrome is an important cause of severe mental and physical handicap in girls. Although normal in early infancy, such girls begin to show evidence of slow psychomotor development towards the end of their first year. Subsequently they have unexplained loss of manipulative skills and speech associated with social withdrawal. Characteristic repetitive hand movements, e.g. hand wringing, rubbing or tapping is a feature of the inexorable decline.

Many progressive neuromuscular diseases of adult life have their onset in childhood. Examples are *myotonic dystrophy* (which may be lethal in the newborn) and *Friedreich's ataxia.*

The floppy infant

Infantile hypotonia is a common problem. Extreme examples are noticed because of paucity of movement, but it is commoner for it to present because of poor head control, floppiness or feeding problems.

When picked up under the arms the baby tends to slip from one's grasp. In ventral suspension the baby flops like a rag doll.

Floppy infants fall into two main groups:

Paralytic

There is severe weakness accompanied by hypotonia. These infants make few movements and may be unable to raise their arm upwards against gravity. It can be caused by a number of rare neuromuscular or spinal cord disorders.

Non-paralytic

More commonly there is hypotonia but only mild weakness. In these babies it is essential to search carefully for the primary condition causing the hypotonia. The possible causes include:
- severe/neurodevelopmental delay
- cerebral palsy—many children who subsequently show spastic diplegia are floppy in early infancy
- certain syndromes—Down's, Prader–Willi
- benign congenital hypotonia. The hypotonia is present in the neonate and may be severe. It does not progress and resolves slowly over several months
- systemic disorders—malnutrition, rickets, hypothyroidism.

OSCE Station: Neurological examination of the legs

Clinical approach:

- observe for other neurological or neuro-developmental problems
- is the child generally alert and aware?
- is she behaving as you would expect?

Gait

- ask mother/child if happy to walk
- best to observe in underwear, no shoes
- observe for:
  ◦ which part of foot strikes floor
  ◦ right and left leg movements
  ◦ symmetry
  ◦ position of rest of body

Inspection

- muscle wasting
- muscle hypertrophy
- asymmetry
- limb shortening
- scars (e.g. lumbosacral, lengthening of TAs)

Tone

- assess tone at hips, knees, and ankles
- don't forget hip adductors and plantarflexors
- clonus

Power

- what does gait and movement tell you?
- power at hip, knee, and ankle

Reflexes

- knee jerks—if absent try reinforcement
- ankle jerks
- plantar response

Beth has difficulty walking. She is 4 years old. Please examine her legs for tone and power

walks with:
- flexed knees and hips
- inturned feet
- toe stepping
- no heel strike

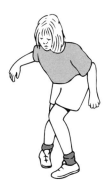

no marks or scars on back

tone ↑ in legs especially:
- hip adductors
→ scissoring
- plantarflexors
→ toe pointing

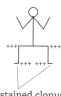

sustained clonus

Beth has spastic cerebral palsy. When legs are affected more than arms, this is a diplegia.

Never forget:

- say hello and introduce yourself
- general health
- colour—?pale/ ?cyanosed
- quickly assess growth, nutrition and development
- mention the obvious (e.g. drip, leg in plaster)

Look around for:

- shoes—Piedro boots
- look at soles of shoes for pattern of wear
- ankle–foot orthoses
- walking aids
- evidence of urinary or faecal problems

Special points

- if the child is willing/ able, begin by asking the child to walk, and then to sit on the floor and get up, **then** use the tendon hammer
- use MRC classification of power if you wish but you do not need to
- show children what you want them to do or give simple explanations

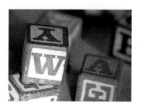

Emotional and Behavioural Problems

Some newborn babies cry often, others are placid: there is no way of knowing whether their different behaviour indicates physical or emotional differences. Sudden loud noises or being dropped may elicit a startled response in newborns, but one cannot tell whether they feel frightened. At 1–2 months the infant begins to become socially responsive, and one can begin to study emotional reactions in infancy.

Social responsiveness is a two-way process and in early life the mother is the vital partner. *Bonding* describes the unique attachment that she develops for her child and which allows her to love, give to, understand and forgive her child. Outwardly it may be manifest by the way in which she holds her child, cuddles, kisses and fondles him, but the all important factor is the ability she has developed to cherish her child through good and bad times. Mothers do not necessarily love their baby at first, it may take several weeks. Ideally parents should be alone with their baby in quiet, happy and untroubled surroundings, but separation, for example by neonatal illness, should not prevent normal attachment.

GOOD PARENTING

- **Positive approach**
  - Praise > criticism
  - Rewards > punishment

- **Discipline**
  - Set limits
  - Constancy
  - Non-victimization
  - Non-oppressive

- **No violence in the home**

- **Opportunities for self development**
  - Encourage learning and exploration
  - Encourage independence

- **Stability**
  - Security within a family home

Probably the most important requirement for healthy emotional development in the early years of life is constancy. A close, personal and physical relationship with one person who provides food, warmth and comfort is an important ingredient. Usually this will be the mother, but it may be the father, grandmother or foster-mother. A child's horizons expand from mother to family to neighbourhood to school and beyond, and at each stage there are new situations to explore and new relationships to establish. Each stage is built on the one before.

Constancy implies that a person, and later a group, can be relied upon to provide the necessities of life, that the person or group is constantly available and does not change and that the responses to exploratory activities are constant. Inconstancy arises: when the child does not know to whom she should turn; when the composition of the home group suddenly changes; the child is removed from it; if she receives conflicting responses, for example, in terms of what she may or may not do. The rules themselves are not so important and will vary from one family to another: but everyone in the family needs to know the rules and to stick to them. In the early months and years the child is putting down his emotional 'roots'. If the ground is forever being disturbed, the roots cannot grow.

The form that an emotional disturbance takes will depend in part upon the cause and in part upon the child's personality and the family patterns of response to stress. Disorders of eating and sleeping usually result from ill-judged or inconsistent handling by parents. Stress is likely to manifest itself as migraine if the child comes from a headache-prone family. The placid child is unlikely to have temper tantrums but may have recurrent abdominal pain. The toddler who feels challenged by the arrival of a new baby may resort to infantile behaviour.

PRESENTATIONS OF EMOTIONAL PROBLEMS

- Psychosomatic disorders — emotional stress causes physical symptoms
- Behavioural disorders

Stress and its symptoms in childhood

The kinds of stress that may precipitate symptoms vary enormously, as does the severity of the stress. Some children are of a buoyant temperament and can ride almost any crisis; others are sensitive plants and bow before every emotional breeze. Some of the stresses most commonly afflicting children are:

Acute separation

The death of a parent or of a much-loved grandparent, emergency admission to hospital or moving house are examples of acute separations. These are most upsetting to young children around 2–4 years old who are conscious of the separation but unable to understand the reason.

Parental discord

All children are conscious of the relationship between their parents and will be aware of any deterioration. When discord develops, the child is likely to be involved and invited to take sides in the contest. This is a devastating experience for all but the most insensitive.

Inconsistent handling

If a child is permitted something by one parent that is denied by the other, or punished on one occasion and ignored on another, this is likely to encourage the more flamboyant kinds of behavioural disorder such as temper tantrums, breath-holding attacks and difficulties with eating and sleeping. The intelligent child is quick to play off one adult against another, or to achieve her own ends by alarming or distressing the adults around her. Diplomacy and blackmail can be learned from an early age.

Boredom

The infant who is deprived of companionship and playthings will be delayed in his development. Without encouragement and practice, motor skills, speech and social activities lag. The bored toddler who is confined to his cot 'to keep him out of mischief', having thrown all toys overboard, can choose between cot rocking, head-banging, pulling out his hair (trichotillomania), masturbating or playing with his excreta. Older children who are bored may take to truancy and vandalism.

Sibling rivalry

Most toddlers, and especially first-borns, delight in the new baby, but may resent the time that their mother devotes to it. If there is regression or aggression, it is likely to be directed against the mother rather than against the baby. When the new baby is old enough to be mobile and to interfere with the elder sibling's activities, jealousy will become more obvious. At school age, constant comparisons between siblings with different capabilities and interests can devastate the less clever or the clumsy. This may lead to antisocial behaviour such as lying, stealing, truancy or wanton destruction.

Great expectations

Parents naturally want their child to do well, but may form an unrealistic idea of her capabilities or set their hearts on a career for her which she could never achieve. Although many a child 'could do better if she tried', not everyone is destined for an honours degree. If parents constantly nag when she is doing her best, psychological breakdown will follow. Recurrent abdominal pain, if it leads to school avoidance, may be the presenting symptom.

Acute emotional shock

Sometimes a child is witness to, or involved in, an acutely distressing situation — a road accident, a sudden death, or sexual abuse. Such an incident may lead to hysterical symptoms (e.g. mutism), to disturbed behaviour (e.g. night terrors), or to acute physical symptoms (e.g. overbreathing).

Stress-related disorders

COMMON PRESENTATIONS

- Recurrent abdominal pain
- Headache
- Vomiting
- Leg ache
- Habit spasms
- Sleep disorders

A large part of clinical practice involves children (and adults) with pains and other symptoms for which no satisfactory cause can be found. Deciding whether the symptoms are secondary to stress can be difficult. Multiple investigations 'to exclude organic disease' are not rewarding and are often unpleasant. History, examination and growth monitoring will usually exclude serious disease. It is rarely helpful to label a pain as psychogenic — which may be interpreted as imagined or fabricated. Better to adopt a comprehensive approach and accept that all symptoms result from the interaction of the body and mind, and that the expression of either physical disorder or good health is modified not only by physical factors, but also intellectual, emotional and social.

After listening to the history, there are two useful supplementary questions, 'What sort of a boy/girl is he/she?' Children with stress symptoms are more often described as nervous, worriers, perfectionists or solitary than as placid, happy-go-lucky or gregarious. 'Who does he take after?' usually elicits a rueful smile and the admission that one or both parents are cast in the same die. This helps understanding. Examination reveals no disease, but bitten fingernails may indicate the tension behind the smile.

Recurrent abdominal pain

Abdominal pain is by far the most common of the stress-related symptoms and it has usually persisted for a year or more by the time medical advice is sought. The pain is almost always central, does not radiate widely and may be associated with nausea. It can be severe, the child becoming quiet and pale. It occurs at any time of day, without obvious precipitating cause, but scarcely ever wakes the child at night. The child may complain of pain several times in a week and then not at all for a month or two. As children with recurrent abdominal pain are usually of school age, the parents often suspect some stress at school. The class teacher, whose report is often helpful, suspects some tension at home and is often right.

Stress headache

It is usually frontal. In most cases, headache is the family stress symptom, and one or both parents will admit to migraine or headaches. Classical unilateral *migraine* is associated with nausea or vomiting; a visual aura is much less common in children than in adults with migraine. Migraine sometimes results from sensitivity to food (chocolate, cheese) or food additives.

Vomiting

Vomiting is intimately connected with the emotions ('I'm sick of it all') but is less common than pain as a stress symptom. It occurs at a younger age than recurrent pains.

Management

It is not to be expected that stress symptoms will be spirited away, but help can be given by the exclusion of organic disease (especially the mythical grumbling appendix), by explanation of the nature of the symptoms and by encouragement not to pay undue attention to them. It is also wise for the doctor to make clear that she understands that the pains are real and not imaginary. Every effort should be made to identify stresses, and health visitors and teachers can be very helpful, but often the symptom is being perpetuated by parental anxiety, in which case a careful history and examination coupled with firm reassurance may be all that is needed.

Enuresis

> The inappropriate voiding of urine at an age when control of micturition would be expected.

Children learn to be dry by day at about 2 years, and by night at about 3 years. By 4 years, 75% of children are dry by day and night. Most children who wet have 'intermittent' enuresis: it is exceedingly rare to encounter children of school age who have never had a dry night. Bed wetting (*nocturnal enuresis*) is a commoner problem than daytime wetting (*diurnal enuresis*).

Nocturnal enuresis

Noctural enuresis is commoner in boys and in lower social classes. Its origins are multiple, and in any child may result from several factors. A genetic predisposition, with a positive family history, is common. Developmental delay may be a factor: just as some children are late walking so some are late at learning to control micturition. Stressful events, like a hospital admission, at the time when the child was learning to be dry may interfere with the learning process and severe stress later in childhood sometimes causes a relapse of enuresis. Most enuretic children do not suffer from either a psychological illness or an organic illness.

- Boys are slower at acquiring dryness than girls
- At the age of 5, over 10% of children wet the bed at least once a week
- At the age of 15, 1% are still wetting the bed

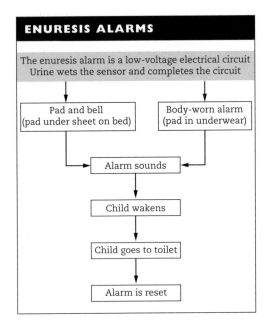

ENURESIS ALARMS

The enuresis alarm is a low-voltage electrical circuit
Urine wets the sensor and completes the circuit

Pad and bell
(pad under sheet on bed)

Body-worn alarm
(pad in underwear)

Alarm sounds

Child wakens

Child goes to toilet

Alarm is reset

Fig. 12.1 Enuresis alarms.

Any condition causing polyuria (e.g. diabetes or renal insufficiency) or bladder irritation (e.g. urine infection) may cause bed wetting, but it is rare for bed wetting to be the presenting symptom of those illnesses. The child with enuresis should have a full physical examination, if only to reassure the parents who may be convinced of his illness. If as is usual the child has had a few nights completely dry, one can be sure that there is no defect in the mechanics of the urinary tract such as ectopic ureter or neuropathic bladder. The urine should be tested for glucose, and for infection.

Management of the enuretic child is a rewarding art. It is a condition that will go, and in most cases an enthusiastic doctor can accelerate the natural cure. Concern and time to listen and explain are vital. Sometimes the home situation, with the mother spending the days washing the sheets and the nights changing them, is so tense that

the general atmosphere of stress and bad temper increases the wetting. Punishment has little place: most children are anxious, indeed over-anxious to stop wetting. Rewards and encouragement may help. The child can be given a notebook, diary or chart in which to stick coloured stars after a dry night. This chart also helps the doctor assess progress. Conditioning therapy by enuresis alarm (Fig. 12.1) is useful for children over the age of 7, and has a high success rate.

Alarms need to be used for 3 or 4 months and require much effort by the child and family, but at the end most children either awaken before they wet (and go to the lavatory), or sleep through without wetting.

Drugs have limited use in the treatment of nocturnal enuresis. Although both the tricyclic antidepressant drugs (e.g. imipramine) and antidiuretics (e.g. desmopressin) reduce bed wetting whilst the drug is being taken, most of those children relapse when the drug is stopped.

Diurnal enuresis (daytime wetting)

Roughly 1% of healthy children over the age of 5 have troublesome daytime wetting; most of them are reliably dry at night. The problem is commoner in girls and is usually the result of *urge incontinence*. (Urodynamic investigation would show bladder instability.) Half the girls who wet by day have recurrent bacteriuria — the bacteriuria contributes to bladder instability and urge incontinence which itself results in damp, smelly pants which predispose to infection. There is an increased incidence of emotional disorder compared with children who merely wet the bed. With increase in age there is a natural tendency to become dry and that acquisition of dryness is accelerated by eradication of bacteriuria and an energetic management regimen which places responsibility on the child voiding more frequently.

Disturbance of bowel habit

Potty training may be started any time in the first 2 years, and a few parents choose to defer it for longer. If started very young, it is the parents who are training themselves to put a pot under the baby when he is going to pass faeces or urine, most commonly after a feed. This helps to establish a conditioned reflex, reinforced by praise when something arrives in the pot but not by punishing the reverse. Toddlers should not be left sitting on their pots for long periods, nor should potty training be obsessional or coercive ('You can't until . . .'). Faulty bowel training predisposes towards constipation which may become life-long.

> ### BOWEL DISTURBANCES
>
> - *Chronic constipation*, which may be complicated by *faecal soiling*
> - *Faecal incontinence* resulting from neurological disorders
> - *Encopresis*: deliberate defaecation in inappropriate places
> - *Toddler diarrhoea* (p. 158).

Faecal soiling, which is most common at 5–10 years, begins as constipation leading to faecal retention. Hard stool causes pain and anal fissure which inhibits defaecation and increases constipation. At other times poor toilet training has resulted in infrequent and incomplete bowel actions. The rectum becomes distended with impacted faeces. In extreme cases, only liquid matter can escape, causing spurious diarrhoea with faecal soiling, of which the child is unaware. His school companions, by contrast, are only too well aware of it, and the child with soiling may become a social outcast.

The abdomen contains hard, faecal masses, often filling the lower half of the abdomen. There is unlikely to be confusion with the rare Hirschsprung's disease, which usually presents at a much earlier age with failure to thrive.

Management involves the thorough emptying of accumulated faeces with laxatives or enemata. Bowel training must then be instituted by regular toileting and the use of faecal softening agents. Laxatives may be needed for several months. The addition of fibre (e.g. bran) to the diet is helpful: ideally the whole family should adopt a high fibre diet. Instant success is not to be expected because the rectum takes time to resume its normal calibre and sensation.

Encopresis is a symptom of serious psychological upset and the advice of a child psychiatrist should be sought.

Habit spasms (tics)

Repetitive, involuntary movements, involving particularly the head and neck, may occur in response to emotional stress. Tics are not rhythmical and cannot be stopped voluntarily. They are most frequent in boys aged 8–11 years. There may have been a reason for the movement initially — a twist of the neck in an uncomfortable collar, a forceful blink because of eyelid irritation — but the movement persists when the reason has gone. Entreaties (or threats) to the child to desist only make it worse and the family are advised to try and overlook the child's irritating habit.

Sleep disorders

Sleepless children demoralize parents. Young children are demanding by day, but parents survive if they can enjoy peaceful nights. Sleeplessness may begin for a good reason, but persist as a bad habit. Children differ in their personalities from birth: some seem to be born 'difficult', while others are 'so easy'.

Young infants sleep most of the time and crying usually indicates hunger, thirst, cold or pain. The infants of anxious or depressed mothers often seem to be tense and cry readily.

The most difficult sleep problems are usually seen in toddlers. Some do not settle down when put to bed: others sleep for a few hours and are then full of activity when the rest of the household is sound asleep. By the time advice is sought these habits have usually persisted for a long time and parents have tried both protracted and complicated bedtime routines, and the almost irreversible step of admitting the child to the parental bed. It is noticeable that whilst the parents often look worn out, the offending child has boundless energy.

Sleep disorders may date from an illness or upset in which a few broken nights were to be expected, but has been protracted by over-solicitous attention. Another common cause is putting the child to bed too early or at no fixed time. Children vary enormously in their sleep requirements and sometimes seem to need less than their parents. If put to bed early, either because they are thought to need so many hours' sleep or because parents like a little time together in the evening, they are wide awake and resent being confined to a cot.

Sleep problems are best prevented by a sensible routine and a firm line when unreasonable demands are made. Before resorting to drugs it is worth trying simple remedies. Is the child is fearful of the dark, a night light or open door to a lit landing may bring calm. If the child demands the presence of mother until asleep, she may accept instead an article of her clothing as a talisman. If bad habits are firmly established, temporary use of hypnotics may be unavoidable.

Nightmares

Bad dreams are common at all ages. Parents, having experienced them themselves, are not usually very worried by them. They know that nightmares occur in normal people and that they do not mean major emotional upset. Measures such as leaving the bedroom door open, or a light on, may comfort the child who is frightened of going to bed. Nightmares occur during rapid eye movement (REM) sleep and are the culmination of a frightening dream adventure, the details of which the child can remember immediately afterwards.

Night terrors

Night terrors are not common, but are most alarming. They occur mainly in the first hour or two of sleep. The child shrieks, sits up and stares wide-eyed and terrified as if being attacked by something only he can see. He may stumble out of bed and seem oblivious to the parents' soothing words. However, within a few minutes he will be sound asleep again and will remember nothing in the morning. Night terrors occur during non-REM sleep, and occur abruptly (not as the result of a dream sequence). They are accompanied by an alarming rise of the pulse and violent respirations which may at times make the parents or doctor suspect an epileptic fit. The parents can be reassured that night terrors do not indicate serious psychological abnormality, and that the child will outgrow them. Gently calming the child back to sleep is all that is needed.

Sleep walking

This may occur independently or as an extension of night terrors, though the sleepwalker tends to be slightly older (e.g. 6–12 years). The child gets out of bed and may walk around the house or even into the street. Although difficult to awaken, he can be guided back to bed. Regardless of that he will usually find his own way back to bed and to sleep. Neither sleep walking nor night terrors should be considered as evidence of major emotional disturbance. Both conditions tend to be familial and to disappear before adolescence.

Crying babies

All normal babies cry. Excessive crying, especially at night, exhausts parents and invites physical abuse. Pain (e.g. earache) may be responsible for short-term crying. Persistent crying more often reflects household tensions. Mothers who seek advice about excessive crying may be afraid that they or their husbands will lose their tempers and damage the baby. The problem may sound trivial to a busy doctor but must *always* be taken seriously. The health visitor can often help.

Breath-holding attacks

Breath-holding attacks are common but harmless; they occur in 1–2% of children up to 3 years, and are precipitated by frustration or pain. After one lusty yell the child holds his breath, goes red in the face, and may later become cyanosed and briefly lose consciousness. He then starts breathing again and is soon back to normal. Sometimes cerebral hypoxia is sufficient to cause brief generalized twitching, and the possibility of epilepsy may then be raised. A careful history will usually resolve any doubts. The attacks are benign and self-limiting. The parents require explanation and reassurance. If they can ignore the attacks, this is ideal. If they feel compelled to action, a little cold water over the head will relieve the tension all round. Sedatives and tranquillizers are not necessary.

The disorders so far described in this chapter lie within the competence of the GP and paediatrician. Help from child psychiatrists and psychologists is usually needed to deal with antisocial behaviour in adolescents and with the more serious behavioural disorders.

Severe behavioural disorders

Anorexia nervosa

This is uncommon in children, but important. It occurs more commonly in girls than in boys, and rarely before puberty. In contrast to children who eat poorly because they are depressed, children with anorexia nervosa appear to have an abundance of energy strangely at variance with their microscopic food intake and steadily falling weight. They look ill but insist that they feel well. It is a serious disease which can be fatal.

Autistic behaviour

- Avoidance of human contact (e.g. eye contact)
- Speech delay
- Obsession with sameness and rituals

Sometimes the onset of symptoms is very early; a mother may say, 'As a baby he would never let me cuddle him'. This sort of behaviour is not uncommon amongst children with learning disorders.

Infantile autism is autistic behaviour in children without other disability, and presents between the 1st and 2nd birthday. Such children are often difficult to handle and always difficult to teach because of their inability to communicate.

Children with less severe autistic behaviour, and normal intelligence, may merely appear odd or eccentric. They are considered to have *Asperger's syndrome* or 'schizoid personality'.

Hyperkinetic behaviour

Children vary greatly in the extent of their activity and concentration and it is impossible to define the limit between physiological and pathological degrees of over-activity. Many normal children are 'always on the go', 'never still', and need relatively few hours of sleep. Beyond this is the hyperkinetic syndrome in which these features interfere with learning or development. In children of school age this presents a grave educational problem.

HYPERKINETIC SYNDROME

- **Inattention**
  - Changes activity frequently
  - Will not persist with tasks

- **Overactivity**
  - Fidgetiness
  - Restlessness

- **Impulsiveness**
  - Impetuous erratic behaviour
  - Frequent accidents
  - Thoughtless rule breaking

The hyperkinetic (hyperactivity) syndrome is more common in boys, and in children with evidence of brain damage, which further complicates their education. Behaviour modification therapy can help. For some, methylphenidate may have a quietening effect, but drug therapy may be difficult to stop. In some children hyperactivity is caused or aggravated by particular foods or (more often) colourings. A properly supervised exclusion diet is worth trying: any improvement in behaviour will be evident within a few days.

Attention deficit disorder may occur with or without hyperactivity. It is often referred to as *attention deficit hyperactivity disorder (ADHD)* and *attention deficit disorder (ADD)*.

OSCE Station: History taking—pain

Clinical approach:

- begin with open questions (e.g. could you tell me what worries you?)
- then focus to more specific questions

Pain

- nature
- site
- first and last occurence
- duration of each episode
- frequency
- length of history
- severity
  - ◇ how bad is it?
  - ◇ can parents tell pain is present?
  - ◇ does it stop him playing/going back to school?
- timing
  - ◇ day/night etc.
  - ◇ school days/holidays
- modifying factors
  - ◇ stress
  - ◇ medicines
  - ◇ food/starvation

Associated symptoms

- vomiting
- diarrhoea/constipation
- enuresis/dysuria
- headache

Gary is 11 years old. His mother is worried about his abdominal pain. He has not been at school for 4 weeks. Please take a brief history

- Mother's biggest worry: Gary is missing time at his new school

- central ache
- most of each day
- not at night
- better at weekends
- appetite good
- sleeping well
- no other symptoms

- Gary's mother is clearly very anxious
- Gary is not present. He spends most of his time watching TV
- no other significant history

Gary has stress-related abdominal pain. It may have been precipitated by the move to a new school. The mother is usually a member of staff who has been given a history

---

Never forget:

- say hello and introduce yourself
- tell the parent(s) and child what you aim to do
- general health—is the child ill?
- ask, is there anything else you think I should know?

If asked or time permits:

- full history
- do not forget
  - ◇ birth history
  - ◇ development
  - ◇ immunizations
  - ◇ family/social history

Look around for:

- family interaction
- parental anxiety
- evidence of care or neglect

Special points

- if exact answer not known (e.g. how long?) ask for approximate answer
- ask if problem is getting better, getting worse, or staying the same
- what do the parents think about the cause of the pain?
- does severity of pain match impact on the child's life (e.g. time off school?)

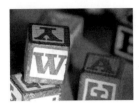

Cardiology

Congenital abnormalities of the heart represent the commonest important group of congenital anomalies. Heart defects occur in nearly 1% of live born infants. An abnormal heart may be found in around 10% of fetuses who are spontaneously aborted. Routine examination of the heart antenatally has led to an increased rate of fetal diagnosis. Most cardiac conditions present as a heart murmur, heart failure or the presence of cyanosis.

The duty of the doctor is to recognize the possibility of heart disease, distinguish it from normal, and assess the urgency of the need for cardiological assessment. This can be difficult.

> Cardiac murmurs do not always mean heart disease.
> Severe heart disease may occur without a murmur.

The cause of congenital abnormalities is usually not known. Environmental factors may be important. These include a congenital viral infection (e.g. rubella, toxoplasmosis) and maternal disease (e.g. diabetes mellitus and systemic lupus erythematosis). Maternal drug therapy during pregnancy (e.g. warfarin, phenytoin or excessive alcohol intake) may lead to congenital heart abnormalities. Recently, a minor abnormality of the 22nd chromosome has been found to be important in children with heart lesions.

In children with isolated congenital heart disease, recurrence risk for subsequent siblings is about 3%. The risk to offspring of a parent with congenital heart disease is 5–10%; 10–20% of children with congenital heart disease have other abnormalities.

Innocent murmurs

CLINICAL FEATURES OF AN INNOCENT MURMUR

- Asymptomatic
- Accentuated by fever/exercise
- Varies with respiration/posture
- Systolic/continuous

These murmurs (also called benign, functional and physiological) occur in children without any cardiac abnormality and are especially common in the newborn. Three main types of innocent murmur are recognized.

Vibratory murmur

This is like the quiet buzzing of a bee. It is very short, mid systolic and less obvious when the child sits up. It usually disappears by puberty.

Pulmonary systolic murmur

This is a soft, blowing ejection systolic murmur, heard at the upper left sternal edge. The differential diagnosis is a mild pulmonary stenosis.

Venous hum

This is due to blood cascading into the great veins. It is a blowing continuous murmur best heard above or below the clavicles. The hum is greatly diminished when the ipsilateral internal jugular vein is compressed, or when the child lies down flat.

Changes in circulation at birth

The changes that take place in the circulation at birth explain why symptoms of congenital heart disease do not occur with some lesions until a few weeks after birth (Fig. 13.1). In the fetus, only 15% of the right ventricular blood enters the lungs, the rest passes through the ductus arteriosus to the descending aorta; the ductus is as large as the aorta. Oxygen levels in the lung tissue are low, pulmonary arteries constrict and, in the fetus, a high pulmonary vascular resistance is maintained.

After birth the following changes take place:

1 Pulmonary interstitial oxygen increases;
2 Pulmonary vascular resistance falls and pulmonary blood flow increases;
3 Systemic vascular resistance rises;
4 The ductus arteriosus closes;
5 The foramen ovale closes.

The fall in pulmonary artery pressure takes place in the first three days of life. The ductus closes within 10–15 h. In lesions with a left to right shunt, the volume of blood shunted increases over the first weeks as pulmonary blood pressure falls.

Congenital heart disease

In Europe, most heart disease in children is congenital. There is a spectrum of severity in each defect from mild to severe and in every lesion changes take place as a child grows, sometimes for better and sometimes for worse. Most severe symptoms occur in the first year of life, particularly in the newborn infant, and urgent investigation and treatment are required. Mild lesions cause no symptoms, are compatible with a normal life and require no treatment. Full initial assessment and follow up is important to prevent secondary changes in the myocardium.

Table 13.1 Congenital heart abnormalities.

CONGENITAL HEART ABNORMALITIES

Condition	Typical heart abnormality
Down's syndrome	Atrioseptal defect
Trisomy 13 or 18	Complex septal defects
Turner's syndrome (45XO)	Coarctation of the aorta
Marfan's syndrome	Aortic aneurysm

PROPHYLAXIS AGAINST ENDOCARDITIS

- Dentistry: extraction, scaling
- Surgery (all operations)
- Invasive non-operative procedure (e.g. endoscopy)

Standard prophylaxis
Amoxycillin: <5 years—750 mg; 5–10 years—1.5 g, >10 years—1.5 g
No general anaesthesia: 1 dose, 1 h before procedure
General anaesthesia: 1 dose 4 h before and one dose soon after procedure

Special precautions—need advice
- Allergy to penicillins
- Antibiotics in previous month
- Previous endocarditis
- Prosthetic valve

CHANGES IN CIRCULATION AT BIRTH

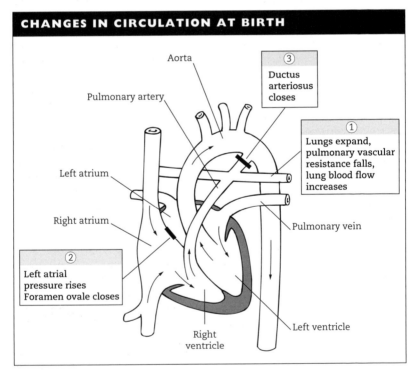

Fig. 13.1 Changes in circulation at birth.

Primary myocardial disease and endocarditis are rare. Rheumatic fever (p. 178) and heart disease are still prevalent in developing countries, but are now rarely seen in Europe.

Neonatal presentations

The symptoms which may occur *should* be explained to the parents of an infant with a heart murmur on discharge. They should be advised to return for early assessment if they are concerned.

Heart murmur

The commonest clinical presentation is the discovery of a heart murmur during routine examination in the first days of life (p. 58). This is an indication for full clinical assessment and a careful search for other congenital abnormalities. If any cardiac symptoms are present, urgent cardiological assessment is indicated. If the infant remains well, but the murmur persists beyond 24–48 h, assessment by an experienced paediatrician or cardiologist is justified. In most paediatric practice, if a murmur is present over the first weeks of life, even if it is thought to be innocent, echocardiography is performed.

Cyanosis

Central cyanosis occurs when the concentration of deoxygenated haemoglobin is greater than 5 g/dL. This must be distinguished from peripheral cyanosis (hands and feet) which is common and normal in the first days of life.

In some infants cyanosis becomes gradually more apparent, while the infant remains otherwise well. This presentation is typical of Fallot's tetralogy (p. 135).

In some infants the presentation is dramatic. The infant is hypoxic, she may be collapsed and acidotic, with a clinical picture which is hard to distinguish from severe infection. A nitrogen washout test may be helpful. The infant is placed in 100% oxygen

for 10–20 min. In severe lung disease, persistent fetal circulation and cyanotic congenital heart disease the blood oxygen does not rise.

In some conditions blood flow to the lungs is dependent on the patent ductus arteriosus. The infant becomes very ill when the ductus closes. The emergency treatment aims to maintain duct patency with prostaglandin. Neonatal intensive care and ventilation is often required. Definitive treatment depends upon diagnosis.

Heart failure

Acute heart failure may occur in left-sided obstructive lesions (e.g. coarctation of the aorta). In such infants, systemic blood flow may depend upon the ductus and prostaglandin may be used.

Over the first weeks of life, increasing left-to-right shunting may produce right sided heart failure of insidious onset with a characteristic set of signs and symptoms (p. 137). In mild failure, these are hard to recognize.

Classification of congenital heart disease

Eight lesions represent 80% of congenital heart disease (Fig. 13.2). Obstructive lesions reduce flow in the outflow tracts or aorta. If the lesion produces a connection between the systemic and pulmonary circulations, a L → R shunt occurs. In the cyanotic lesions, there is obstruction to the pulmonary circulation (e.g. Fallot) or abnormal circulation (e.g. transposition of the great arteries).

Diagnosis

Initially assessment is by clinical examination. Chest X-ray and ECG are helpful, but the most important diagnostic tool is echocardiography with Doppler assessment, which allows estimation of flow. Only rarely is cardiac catheterisation required. Full assessment of non-cardiac problems

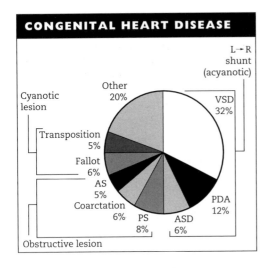

CONGENITAL HEART DISEASE

Fig. 13.2 Classification of congenital heart disease.

can be critically important if major surgery is being considered.

Left-to-right shunts

Ventricular septal defect (VSD)
The natural history of VSD depends upon the size of the defect, the changes that occur with growth, and the behaviour of the pulmonary circulation.

Small defects
Patients have no symptoms and the heart murmur is heard during routine examination. 75% close in the first 10 years of life (the majority by 2 years) but closure goes on occurring in adult life. The only risk is of bacterial endocarditis.

Medium-sized defects
These cause symptoms in infancy. Heart failure results in poor feeding and slow weight gain. Symptoms appear in the first months of life, often precipitated by a chest infection. Improvement occurs following medical treatment. As the child grows, the defect becomes relatively smaller, symptoms lessen, and weight gain improves. Closure usually occurs.

Large defects
Symptoms begin in the first weeks of life. Heart failure is difficult to control and tube feeding is necessary. A small number close, but most need surgery. In infancy, persistent high pulmonary blood flow leads to increased pulmonary vascular resistance. The volume of the L → R shunt diminishes and heart failure improves. It is important not to be misled by this apparent improvement, because if the defect is not closed before the age of 2 years, changes in the lung vessels become permanent. Without surgery, pulmonary vascular disease worsens, the shunt reverses, the patient becomes cyanosed and breathless and will die in the second or third decade. The only management of pulmonary vascular disease is prevention with early surgery.

Signs

Turbulent blood flow from the left to the right ventricle causes a pan-systolic murmur at the left sternal edge, maximal in the third and fourth left interspaces. Loud murmurs cause a systolic thrill.

Treatment

Medical treatment (e.g. diuretics, ACE inhibitors) is used to control the heart failure. The defect is closed surgically using cardiopulmonary bypass if symptoms cannot be controlled or there is a danger of pulmonary vascular disease developing.

Patent ductus arteriosus (PDA)

PDA is most common in the preterm infant. Murmur and heart failure are noted in the first weeks during intensive care, and it may be difficult to reduce the infant's ventilation requirements. Control of heart failure may be sufficient. Some preterm infants require duct closure medically, using indomethacin as a prostaglandin inhibitor, or by surgical ligation. Spontaneous closure occurs up to 3 months after birth.

In the term infant, if the ductus is patent during the first 2 weeks of life, spontaneous closure is rare. A large PDA leads to heart failure, and in others the persisting risk of bacterial endarteritis is an indication for surgical closure.

Signs

The pulses are collapsing because of the sudden leak of blood from the aorta to the pulmonary artery. The characteristic finding is a continuous, 'machinery' (systolic and diastolic) murmur under the left clavicle (Fig. 13.3). There may be a thrill.

Treatment

Heart failure is treated medically. If the ductus remains patent, closure is indicated. A duct may be ligated at surgery, or occluded with a small 'double umbrella' device which is placed in the ductus through a cardiac catheter.

HEART MURMURS

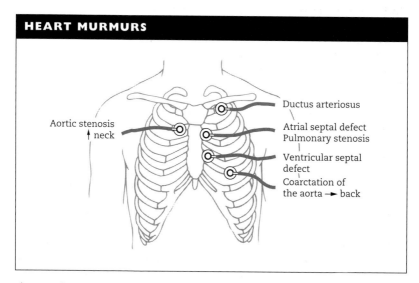

Fig. 13.3 The murmur is heard loudest at the point shown. Some loud murmurs can be heard over the whole precordium. Some murmurs radiate in a characteristic direction.

Atrial septal defect (ASD)

ASD does not usually cause symptoms in childhood because the L → R shunt is small. In the majority a heart murmur is discovered during routine examination and the child has few or no symptoms. Symptoms occur in the second and third decades, pulmonary hypertension develops secondary to the large blood flow into the lungs, and heart failure and atrial dysrhythmias result.

Signs

There is a right ventricular heave due to increased blood volume. An ejection systolic murmur is heard in the pulmonary area due to excessive blood flow through a normal pulmonary valve. The second heart sound is widely split because it takes longer for the volume overloaded right ventricle to empty and the pulmonary valve closure is delayed. The wide splitting does not vary with respiration and is described as 'fixed' (p. 34). The chest X-ray shows pulmonary plethora.

Treatment

Atrial septal defects should be closed surgically by school age to prevent late pulmonary hypertension.

Obstructive lesions

Coarctation of aorta

Severe coarctation

If severe, acute symptoms occur in the neonatal period. Blood flows through the patent ductus arteriosus from the pulmonary artery to the lower half of the body. When the duct closes, the left ventricle cannot maintain the flow of blood to the aorta and left and right ventricular failure results. Unless treatment is given urgently, the child dies.

Signs

The baby is breathless, grey and collapsed with hepatomegaly. The pulses are better in the arms than the legs but may be difficult to feel everywhere. Blood pressure is lower in the legs than the arms. There are no murmurs.

Treatment

Prostaglandin E is given to re-open the ductus. Heart failure is controlled prior to urgent surgery. The ductus is ligated and the coarctation repaired.

Mild coarctation

These children often have no symptoms and gradually a collateral circulation develops. Hypertension occurs in the head and arms. Without surgery, most would die in their 30s and 40s.

Signs

The pulses in the arms and neck are normal. Femoral and leg pulses are delayed, weak or absent. The blood pressure is raised in the arms, but lower in the legs. There may be a systolic murmur best heard between the shoulder blades.

> The key to detection of coarctation of the aorta is routine examination of the femoral pulses.

Treatment

Surgery is advised in all patients as soon as the diagnosis is made.

Aortic stenosis (AS)

Most children with mild stenosis have no symptoms and no restriction of exercise is necessary. In adult life valve calcification occurs and the stenosis becomes more severe. In severe stenosis, syncope and dizziness are the first symptoms, and the risk of sudden death is 1%. In the severe group, stressful exercise may cause symptoms or even angina and is avoided. In critical (very severe) stenosis, heart failure occurs in the first weeks of life, and if AS is not recognized 50% die. The severity of the stenosis is assessed by measuring the pressure gradient across the valve using Doppler echocardiography. Prevention of endocarditis is very important.

Signs
An ejection systolic murmur is best heard in the aortic area and conducted to the neck. There may be an ejection click. Systolic thrills occur in the suprasternal notch and over the right carotid artery. ECG shows left ventricular hypertrophy.

Treatment
Most children with significant AS eventually will need valve replacement. In childhood, surgery is palliative, and aims to delay valve replacement. Balloon dilatation may be used to relieve stenosis.

Pulmonary stenosis (PS)
Most pulmonary stenosis is mild, will not affect a child's health, and is unlikely to worsen during the patient's lifetime. In more severe stenosis, although there may be no symptoms, the stenosis becomes relatively greater as the patient grows and progressive hypertrophy of the right ventricular muscle occurs. Eventually there is a limitation of cardiac output, and breathlessness, dysrhythmias and heart failure occur. Critical pulmonary stenosis in infancy will cause early death unless recognized, and may present dramatically when the ductus arteriosus closes.

Signs
A loud ejection systolic murmur occurs in the second left interspace. There may be a thrill. The murmur radiates backwards. There is a right ventricle heave and wide splitting of the second sound. ECG shows right ventricular hypertrophy.

Treatment
Balloon dilatation or surgery is used to relieve severe stenosis.

Cyanotic lesions

Tetralogy of Fallot
Most children with Fallot's present in the first month of life with a murmur and the gradual onset of cyanosis (Fig. 13.4). Surprisingly, cyanosis may be difficult to detect and far from obvious. The classical picture of cyanosis at rest and on exertion, in the child who squats in order to increase pulmonary blood flow, is now avoided by surgery.

Children with Fallot's develop cyanotic attacks. Without warning, the child cries in pain, becomes breathless and cyanosed, and may lose consciousness fleetingly. Such attacks may be dangerous and recognition of a typical history is important.

Children with Fallot's are at risk of myocardial infarction, cerebral vascular accidents, endocarditis, embolus and cerebral abscess.

Signs
Without surgery, children are cyanosed with clubbing. There is a right ventricle heave and a systolic murmur at the upper left sternal edge due to the narrowed right ventricular outflow tract. Cardiac failure does not occur.

X-ray
Right ventricular hypertrophy: boot-shaped heart.

Treatment
Cyanotic attacks are treated with oxygen, β-blocker and analgesia.

Corrective surgery is usually performed within the first year. In infants with severe early symptoms, a temporary anastomosis is created between the subclavian artery

FALLOT'S TETRALOGY

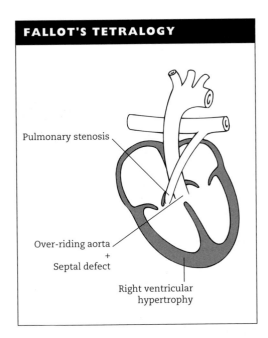

Pulmonary stenosis

Over-riding aorta
+
Septal defect

Right ventricular
hypertrophy

Fig. 13.4 Fallot's tetralogy.

and the pulmonary artery to increase pulmonary blood flow.

Transposition of the great arteries (TGA)

TRANSPOSITION OF THE GREAT ARTERIES

- Two independent parallel circulations

- Oxygenated pulmonary venous blood
  → pulmonary artery

- De-oxygenated systemic venous blood
  → aorta

- Mixing of two circulations
  ◆ Atrial septum
  ◆ Ductus arteriosus
  ◆ VSD

In transposition, there must be a connection between the two parallel circulations to allow some mixing, or the condition is incompatible with life. Transposition presents acutely in the first days of life, as the cyanosis increases and the ductus arteriosus closes. The child becomes breathless, unable to feed, and may be extremely ill. There may or may not be a murmur.

X-ray
The heart has a narrow pedicle and is like an egg with the pointed part of the egg forming the apex of the heart ('egg on its side').

Treatment
Unless urgent treatment is given, these children die. Prostaglandin is given to maintain patency of the ductus arteriosus. The emergency treatment is balloon septostomy. A cardiac catheter is passed through the atrial septum. A balloon on the end is then inflated and pulled back sharply into the right atrium in order to tear the atrial septum.

This allows mixing of blood between the two atria.

Surgical correction is now performed in the first months of life. In the arterial switch procedure, the aorta and pulmonary artery are divided above the valves and switched over.

Surgical treatment of congenital heart disease

As cardiac surgery advances there is a tendency to operate on the common lesions earlier in life. This often means operating before the child has any symptoms. Surgery is generally safe, with operative mortality less than 5%. In a large majority, long-term myocardial function is normal.

INFORMING PARENTS ABOUT HEART DISEASE

- Parents are shocked to hear their child has heart disease
- Cause is usually unknown—it is not their fault
- Congenital heart disease is not like ischaemic heart disease
- Exercise restriction is hardly ever necessary (except in severe aortic stenosis).
- Try to provide written information and a diagram
- Echocardiography (cardiac ultrasound) is the important early investigation
- Not all congenital heart disease requires surgery
- Prophylaxis against endocarditis is important.

Cardiac failure

Heart failure is a medical emergency. It occurs more commonly in the first 3 months of life than in any other period of childhood

and is usually due to congenital heart disease (Fig. 13.5). Earlier onset implies a more severe heart lesion. It is also caused by myocarditis and endocarditis.

CLINICAL FEATURES OF HEART FAILURE

- Poor feeding
- Breathless on exertion
- Sweating
- Poor weight gain
- Excess weight gain (oedema)

Prompt treatment is essential:
- prop the child up and give oxygen
- correct acidosis, hypoglycaemia, hypocalcaemia or anaemia
- treat respiratory infection with antibiotics
- feed by nasogastric tube
- medication: diuretics are important; Frusemide is often combined with spironolactone to prevent potassium loss. Systemic vascular resistance and the work of the left ventricle can be reduced with a vasodilator (e.g. ACE inhibitor).

Dysrhythmias

Abnormalities of sinus rhythm are not usually of cardiac origin. Bradycardia means hypoxia. A tachycardia is often seen in association with fever, dehydration or any acute illness. If episodic dysrhythmia is suspected from the history, ambulatory 24h ECG monitoring can be extremely helpful.

Supraventricular tachycardia (SVT)

SVT is the commonest symptomatic dysrhythmia in childhood. It may rarely occur *in utero* and is controlled by treating the mother. Infants with SVT become

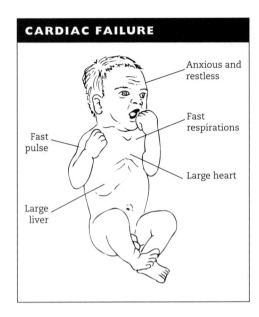

Fig. 13.5 Cardiac failure in infancy.

acutely ill, collapsed and grey and need urgent help.

The pulse is very fast, too fast to count. ECG shows a narrow complex tachycardia (greater than 250 beats per minute).

A child with SVT should be given oxygen and may require intensive care. Vagal stimulation (facial immersion in iced water or the application of an ice bag) is occasionally effective. Rapid intravenous injection of adenosine is usually successful. Some children require long-term treatment to prevent recurrence.

Ventricular extrasystoles

In childhood, extrasystoles are not uncommon and usually of no significance. If there are symptoms or multiple extra systoles, investigation and treatment are required.

Congenital heart block

Heart block may lead to stillbirth. It is usual-ly associated with maternal lupus antibody. Most infants are asymptomatic, but occasionally a pacemaker is necessary.

Hypertension

Measuring blood pressure is not difficult in children. The correct size cuff must be used (see p. 35), and in all but the smallest infants, reliable measurements may be obtained using automated auscultation methods (e.g. Dinamap). In school age children, auscultation is used. A child's blood pressure must be considered against age-related reference values.

In general those children who have a blood pressure about the 90th centile in early life tend to remain at that end of the distribution curve in later childhood and probably adult life also. The blood pressure of any child has a close correlation with that of the parents and siblings.

CAUSES OF HYPERTENSION

- Renal disease
  - Glomerulonephritis
  - Pyelonephritis
  - Congenital defect
  - Renal artery stenosis

- Endocrine
  - Steroid therapy
  - Phaeochromocytoma, congenital adrenal hyperplasia

- Coarctation of the aorta

- Essential

Compared with adults, a primary cause is found more often and, if treated surgically (e.g. unilateral kidney disease or coarctation), may abolish hypertension, some 10–15% have essential hypertension and a cause is not found.

Hypertension may be asymptomatic, or may present in a wide variety of ways: failure to thrive, fits, encephalopathy, retinopathy, heart failure or, in the older child, headaches and malaise. Diuretics and hypotensive drugs are used as for adults — and tolerated rather better by most children.

OSCE Station: Examination of the cardiovascular system

Clinical approach:

Check hands
- clubbing
- colour
- perfusion

Check face
- colour
- anaemia
- respiratory distress

Pulses
- rate
- rhythm
- both radials, and a brachial
- femorals? brachio-femoral delay
- is character of pulses clearly abnormal?

Chest

Inspection
- scars
  ◇ remember under arms and on back

Palpation
- localize apex
- parasternal heave
- palapable thrill

Auscultation
- is heart louder on left?
- two heart sounds
- ?loud P2 ?split second sound

Murmurs
- loudness/quality
- localization
- radiation
- timing

George is 4 years old. Please examine his cardiovascular system

- normal inspection:
  ◇ no scars + no symptoms (this narrows it down!)
  ◇ not cyanosed (so, no R→L shunt)
- pulses normal, femorals ✓✓ normal blood pressure (e.g. 85/55)

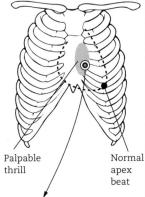

↑ No radiation to neck

Palpable thrill

Normal apex beat

- lower left sternal edge
- 3rd–4th intercostal space
- loud, harsh murmur
- pansystolic

George has an asymptomatic ventricular septal defect.

Never forget:

- say hello and introduce yourself
- general health—is the child breathless?
- colour—?pale/ ?cyanosis
- quickly assess growth, nutrition, and development
- mention the obvious (e.g. drip, leg in plaster)

Look around for:

- nasogastric tube
- pulse oximeter

Special points

- blood pressure and pulse vary with age
- use correct BP cuff size and tell the child what you are doing
- timing a murmur is difficult in young children—most are systolic
- do not suggest Fallot's in a pink 13 year old with no scars
- cardiovascular mal-formations are more common in some syndromes (e.g. Down's)

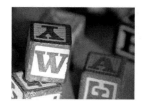

Respiratory Medicine

Respiratory infections and asthma are
major causes of morbidity and are common
reasons for a child being taken to a doctor
or admitted to hospital.

> **i** Recurrent wheeze occurs in over
> 10% of children. The prevalence of mild
> and moderate asthma has increased.

Certain problems are more common at
certain ages and the same organism may
cause different illnesses at different ages.
For example, respiratory syncytial virus
(RSV) commonly causes lower respiratory
tract illness (bronchiolitis) in infants, and a
cold or a sore throat in older children.

Symptoms of respiratory tract disease

Cough in children is usually upper respiratory tract infection (URTI) and less often
lung disease. Distinguish between 'throaty'
and 'chesty' coughs; a barking cough suggests a laryngeal or tracheal disorder (Table
14.1). Young asthmatics may cough instead
of wheeze, especially at night. Children usually swallow their sputum unless it is copious. Purulent and blood stained sputum are
rare.

In acute otitis media, earache is severe,
but it also occurs in many URTIs. Pain from
lower back teeth may be referred to the ear.

RESPIRATORY DISTRESS AND FAILURE

Recognition of severe respiratory disease is essential. Intervene before respiratory
distress leads to respiratory failure.

Respiratory distress (increased work of breathing)
- Tachypnoea (>50/min infants; >40/min in children)
- Intercostal/subcostal recession
- Use of accessory muscles (arms and shoulders)
- Expiratory grunting in infants

Respiratory failure (respiratory effort insufficient or unsustainable)
- Severe respiratory distress or
- Diminished respiratory effort, apnoea
- CNS signs of hypoxia: agitation; fatigue; drowsiness
- Cyanosis
- Collapse.

RESPIRATORY INFECTIONS

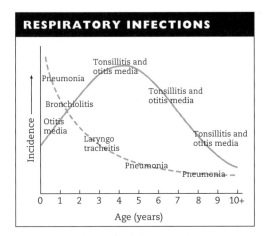

Fig. 14.1 The incidence of respiratory infections.

RESPIRATORY TRACT OBSTRUCTION

Table 14.1 Respiratory tract obstruction.

Stridor (p. 155)	Wheeze
Larynx/trachea	Bronchi/bronchioles
Inspiratory	Expiratory
Monophonic	Polyphonic

Upper respiratory tract

Most illnesses of childhood are infections; most childhood infections are respiratory; most are upper respiratory tract infection (URTI). The great majority are viral. Examination of the ears, nose and throat is mandatory in all febrile children. Tonsillitis and otitis media imply clear evidence of inflammation of the tonsils or middle ears, respectively. An inflamed throat is called pharyngitis.

URTI is used to describe the common cold. The symptoms are cough, anorexia and fever. In the infant nasal obstruction may lead to feeding difficulties. Eustachian tube obstruction often causes earache and the eardrums may appear congested. Antibiotics are not indicated. Paracetamol will reduce fever and relieve discomfort.

URTI may precipitate febrile convulsions (p. 104), and asthma attacks and is sometimes the precursors of acute specific fevers, especially measles (p. 221) or bronchiolitis.

Recurrent coughs and colds

PERSISTENT COUGH

Common
- Chronic rhinorrhoea
- Postnasal drip
- Asthma (exercise, night)
- Cigarette smoke
- Habit

Uncommon
- Pertussis
- Foreign body
- Gastro-oesophageal reflux
- Cystic fibrosis
- Tuberculosis.

Recurrent coughs and colds, sometimes with sore throat and earache, are very common in young children. Some babies and toddlers are catarrhal much of the time. The first winter at school or nursery is frequently punctuated by upper respiratory infections.

Poor social circumstances and passive smoking predispose to catarrh. Some children will not blow their noses; some with severe nasal obstruction cannot. Decongestants and cough suppressants are widely used and variably successful. The best healer is the passage of time.

Apnoea

Temporary cessation of breathing is a frightening occurrence. It can result from central respiratory depression or from mechanical obstruction (including the inhalation of food or vomit). It may occur during the first day or two of respiratory infections, particularly pertussis or respiratory syncytial virus. However, many infants are rushed to hospital by their parents, who believe their child has stopped breathing. Often it is not clear whether anxious parents have merely misinterpreted the normal variable breathing of a small baby, or whether the baby genuinely has had a significant spell of apnoea. When the apnoea is associated with cyanosis, or unconsciousness, the differential diagnosis must include a seizure, congenital heart disease, or airways obstruction. For very worried parents the loan of an apnoea alarm, which sounds when the baby stops breathing, may be comforting. There is no evidence that apnoea alarms prevent sudden infant death syndrome (p. 240). Most children who die suddenly and unexpectedly in early life have not had previous spells of apnoea.

Influenza

Influenza tends to occur in epidemics, affecting particularly school children and young adults. The general symptoms of high fever, headache and malaise tend to overshadow the dry cough and sore throat, though there may be signs of pharyngitis, tracheitis or bronchitis. The main complications result from secondary bacterial infection of lungs, middle ear or sinuses.

The brief incubation period and high infectivity favour massive outbreaks. Immunization against commoner strains is given to children at risk of severe infection. Treatment is symptomatic.

Lower respiratory tract

The bronchial tree and its blood supply are present by the 20th week of gestation, and thereafter only enlarge. In contrast, the alveoli increase in number from 20 million at birth to the adult complement of 300 million. Respiratory disease in early childhood may therefore interfere with future lung development as well as cause direct lung damage. Small airways obstruct or collapse early leading to poor oxygenation or collapse of a lung segment.

Bronchitis

Acute bronchitis occurs at all ages and is characterized by cough, fever and often wheezing. It is a common feature of influenza and whooping cough. Chronic bronchitis does not occur in children.

Bronchiolitis

Bronchiolitis is the commonest cause of severe respiratory infection in infancy; 70% is due to the respiratory syncytial virus (RSV), 90% of children are immune to this virus by 2 years of age. Most children remain at home with this infection but 1–2% of all infants are admitted each year, usually during the winter epidemics.

BRONCHIOLITIS

- Initial coryza
- Cough
- Respiratory distress
- Irritability
- Poor feeding
- Widespread wheeze and crepitations
- Hyperinflated chest.

Younger infants and those with marked respiratory distress are more likely to need hospital admission. Supportive management includes skilled nursing, intravenous fluids, nasogastric feeding and oxygen usually monitored with pulse oximetry. Nasogastric feeding is needed frequently to maintain fluid and calorie intake. Antibiotics are often given if bacterial infection cannot be excluded. The RSV may be detected by fluorescent antibody test on nasopharyngeal secretions.

Most infants recover within a few days. Up to half of infants with RSV bronchiolitis subsequently develop recurrent wheezing.

Pneumonia

Bronchopneumonia

This is commonest in young children and in older children with a chronic condition affecting respiratory function (e.g. cystic fibrosis, severe cerebral palsy). A wide variety of organisms can be responsible. It commonly follows bronchiolitis, viral infection and whooping cough. Clinical features include rapid breathing, dry cough, fever and fretfulness. Generalized crepitations and rhonchi are usually present.

Cyanosis occurs in severe cases and infants may develop cardiac failure. Chest X-ray often shows small patches of consolidation.

Hospitalization is usually needed. Oxygen and a broad-spectrum antibiotic are given. Gentle physiotherapy helps to mobilize secretions. Infants may need tube feeding.

Lobar pneumonia

Pneumonia presents with sudden illness and high fever. The child is sick, looks flushed, breathes fast and has respiratory

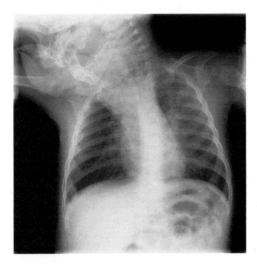

Fig. 14.2 Chest X-ray showing right upper lobe collapse and consolidation.

distress (p. 141). There may be no cough. Pleuritic pain may cause the child to lean towards the affected side, or may be referred to the abdomen or neck. The clinical signs of consolidation may not be present at first, but repeated examination will usually reveal them. A transient pleural rub is common. Lobar consolidation, with or without pleural effusion, is usually evident on X-ray (Fig. 14.2).

PNEUMONIA: CAUSATIVE AGENTS

- *Streptococcus pneumoniae*
- *Mycoplasma pneumoniae*
- *Haemophilus influenzae*
- *Staphylococcus aureus*
- *Mycobacterium tuberculosis*

Lobar pneumonia is usually caused by *Strep. pneumoniae* and penicillin achieves dramatic improvement within 24 h. In the ill child the causative organism is not known initially and broad spectrum antibiotics are used. At least the initial dose of antibiotics is given by injection, as an ill child is likely to vomit medicine. Not all children are severely ill and some can be treated at home. Fluid intake is more important than food. Paracetamol and tepid sponging will help reduce fever.

If improvement does not occur, or if signs or symptoms are still present after a week, careful examination including chest X-ray should be repeated to exclude complications such as pleural effusion of lobar collapse. In the older child particularly, mycoplasma should be considered. The possibility of *tuberculosis* should never be forgotten.

Staphylococcal pneumonia is a severe form of lung infection which usually affects young children and those with chronic predisposing disease. It is characterized by lung cysts on X-ray and the sudden appearance of empyema or pneumothorax. Prolonged treatment is required with an antistaphylococcal antibiotic.

Inhaled foreign bodies

Toddlers are most at risk because they tend to put everything into their mouths. Older children sometimes accidentally inhale objects during games or whilst stuffing their mouths too full of peanuts or sweets.

A foreign body may lodge at any level. At the time the child will cough, splutter or make choking noises but the episode is quickly forgotten and may not come out in the history without specific questioning. In the larynx an object is likely to cause a croupy cough and stridor. If it passes through the larynx, it will lodge in a bronchus (right middle lobe or a lower lobe most often) and there will be no symptoms for a few days until infection, collapse or obstructive emphysema develop.

If a foreign body is suspected, radiography may demonstrate it (if it is radio-opaque) or show associated changes. Diagnosis may require direct laryngoscopy and bronchoscopy, which will be required to remove the object.

The wheezy child

ⓘ Annual deaths from asthma have halved in the last 15 years but 20 children die each year in the UK.

Wheezing is an obstructive respiratory sound arising in the smaller branches of the bronchial tree: on auscultation, rhonchi can be heard. They are most marked in expiration because the bronchial tree dilates in inspiration.

Wheezing is most common in young infants. Some have recurrent episodes limited to the first 2 years. In others, recurrent bouts of wheezing lead to the diagnosis of asthma.

Asthma

ASTHMA

Intermittent, reversible obstruction of the small airways
- Recurrent bouts of wheezing
- Breathlessness and cough.

It is important to try to understand the underlying factors in each wheezy child if the best help is to be given. In young children, upper respiratory tract infections appear to be the commonest precipitating factor, but as the child grows up others may become apparent: specific allergens, exercise, emotional upsets and changes of weather or environment (Fig. 14.3).

Infection
Viral infection is a common precipitant of asthma: Infection is likely to be important in children who have most trouble in winter.

Allergy
Allergens can be best identified from the history (e.g. after specific exposure or in the pollen season). A family history of allergies is common. Specific antibody tests add little to management.

Atopy
Atopy is an IgE-mediated immune response to common environmental antigens. It has a strong genetic basis and commonly manifests as asthma, eczema and/or hay fever in the family.

Emotions
Exceptionally, a severe emotional upset may precipitate a first attack of wheezing. Commonly, excitement or anxiety can precipitate or aggravate attacks.

Exercise
Exercise-induced wheezing occurs most readily when running in a cold atmosphere. Beware the child who can begin a game of football but not last longer than 20 min. Many asthmatics become wheezy on exertion, especially if it involves running.

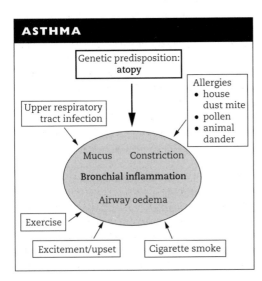

Fig. 14.3 The pathogenesis of asthma.

ASTHMA

History	Examination	Investigation
Acute		
What do child/parents think?	Level of respiratory distress	Oxygen saturation
Therapy received	Tachycardia	Blood gas—abnormalities occur late
Can child run/walk/ drink/talk?	Altered conscious level (drowsy or irritable)	Chest X-ray—if severe
	Beware silent chest (↓ Air entry in severe attack)	PEFR—unreliable in acute attack
Chronic		
Child/parent opinion	Growth	Serial PEFR
Current therapy	Chest shape	Spirometry
Hospital admission	↑ AP diameter	
Lifestyle changes	Harrison's sulci	
Sport		
School attendance		
PEFR, peak expiratory flow rate.		

Table 14.2 History, examination and investigation of asthma.

Atmosphere

Dusty air, 'stuffy' and smoke-filled rooms, or changes in air temperature may precipitate wheezing.

Assessing severity of asthma

(Table 14.2)

Management

The aim is to reduce the frequency and severity of attacks and to give the child and family confidence that they can cope with attacks without disruption of home or school life. Precipitating factors should be sought. In all cases it is worth reducing the child's exposure to common allergens.

> **i**
> Normal peak expiratory flow rate is related to height, not age.
> PEFR = [(height above 100 cm) × 5 + 100] ± 100 L/min (Fig. 14.4)

Those at home are advised not to smoke in the house, particularly in the child's bed-room. Emotional problems at home or school can often be helped, but asthma generates its own emotional problems for the family. It can be a frightening condition. Some children react to animal fur or dander, and occasionally it is necessary for the family pet to be removed.

In some children the history of asthma is obvious. In others, colds 'go to the chest', cough persists and the parents may not notice the wheezing. Typically, the asthmatic child will have recurrent respiratory infections which last longer than her siblings. Night time symptoms of poor sleeping or cough should raise suspicions. It is so common that it should always be sought on direct inquiry in every paediatric history.

Administration of therapy

Whenever possible, asthma therapy should be given by inhalation (Fig. 14.5). In children of school age, dry powder inhalers or metered dose aerosol inhalers (MDI) with a spacer device may be used. All aerosol agents are more effective through a spacer

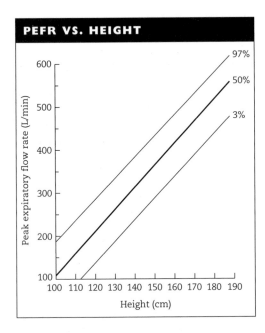

Fig. 14.4 Normal peak expiratory flow rate and height.

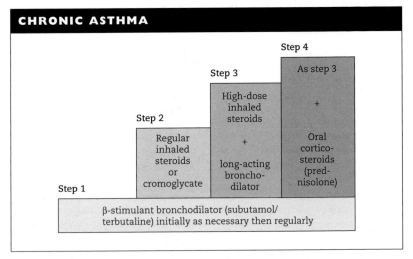

Fig. 14.5 Stepwise approach to chronic asthma. Step up if control is poor and back down when good control is maintained.

device, avoiding the need to synchronize inhalation with the aerosol and improving distribution of the drug in the bronchial tree. In most younger children, a meter dose inhaler with spacer device fitted with a face mask may be used with instruction. This technique can be used in young infants. Nebulized therapy can be given with a little cooperation on the part of the child. It is always best to ask the parent or child to hold the face mask. This is particularly valuable during acute attacks for delivery of β bronchodilators.

Oral therapy with salbutamol or terbutaline is much less effective and side-effects are more likely. Occasionally, oral steroids and xanthines (e.g. theophylline) are necessary in children with severe chronic disease. Oral prednisolone may be given in a short course over a few days to bring about resolution of an acute severe attack.

The commonest reason for poor control in chronic asthma is poor compliance. If control deteriorates abruptly, make sure the family have not just acquired a dog.

> **i** Early, adequate prophylaxis may reduce likelihood of later, severe disease.

Acute severe attacks

ACUTE SEVERE ASTHMA

- Oxygen by face mask
- Nebulized salbutamol with oxygen
- Oral prednisolone

Severe attack not responding
- Intravenous aminophylline
- Intravenous hydrocortisone
- Parenteral β bronchodilator

Children and their families should be taught to recognize acute severe attacks. Worrying features include failure to respond to usual therapy, exhaustion, severe respiratory distress (Table 14.2) and persistent symptoms. Any child who is too breathless to talk or feed, any change in conscious level or any history of colour change or cyanosis implies life threatening illness.

Anyone who has had an asthma attack knows how frightening this can be: calm reassurance to the child and her parents is important. This should not replace the need for urgent assessment and therapy. Most respond to inhaled β bronchodilation. If a nebuliser is not available, repeated doses of

an MDI may be given with the spacer device. The usual dose may be given repeatedly at 30–60 second intervals.

Intravenous therapy with β stimulant, hydrocortisone or aminophylline is reserved for children with severe signs. Aminophylline infusion must always be given slowly and great care should be used if a child is on maintenance theopylline therapy. Supportive therapy with fluids is important. Primary bacterial infections are uncommon, but antibiotics are normally given in severe attacks. Acute sudden deterioration should raise the suspicion of pneumothorax.

Every admission to hospital or outpatient visit should be used as an opportunity to review longer term therapy. No child should be given inhaled therapy without being taught how to use it by an expert. It is important to watch a child using their inhalers and to examine their technique from time to time.

Cystic fibrosis

Cystic fibrosis (CF) is the commonest, lethal inherited condition amongst Europeans. It is an autosomal recessive condition due to mutations of the gene on the seventh chromosome which codes for the cystic fibrosis transmembrane regulator — a protein which controls chloride transport across the cell membrane. Hundreds of mutations have now been found. In the UK around 80% of mutations are a single amino-acid abnormality known as ∆F508. Asymptomatic carriers are 1:25 of the population. CF effects 1:2500 children in the UK.

Clinical features and presentation
The common presentations of CF are:
- Fetal screening (mutation analysis);
- Neonatal screening (genetic or immune — reactive trypsin);

- Neonatal meconium ileus;
- Recurrent respiratory infections;
- Failure to thrive with fatty diarrhoea.

In the newborn baby, meconium may be so glutinous with viscid mucus that normal peristaltic waves cannot shift it (*meconium ileus*). Small amounts of meconium may be passed: generalized abdominal distension and vomiting develop over 24–48 h. Abdominal X-ray shows obstruction. Obstruction may be relieved by careful administration of a water-soluble hyperosmolar enema. Often surgery is necessary. Obviously, all children with meconium ileus must be tested for CF.

Most of the unscreened children with CF

present in childhood. CF should be considered with any combination of the cardinal symptoms. Malabsorption is due to deficiency of pancreatic enzymes and may start any time from birth. Distension and weight loss resemble coeliac disease. *Staphylococcus aureus, haemophilus influenzae* and later *pseudomonas* chest infections, leads to lung

CARDINAL SYMPTOMS OF CF

- Recurrent chest infection
- Loose, offensive stools
- Failure to thrive.

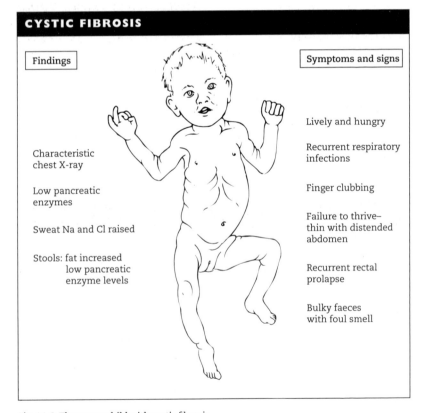

CYSTIC FIBROSIS

Findings

Characteristic chest X-ray

Low pancreatic enzymes

Sweat Na and Cl raised

Stools: fat increased
low pancreatic
enzyme levels

Symptoms and signs

Lively and hungry

Recurrent respiratory infections

Finger clubbing

Failure to thrive—thin with distended abdomen

Recurrent rectal prolapse

Bulky faeces with foul smell

Fig. 14.6 The young child with cystic fibrosis.

damage and bronchiectasis. Untreated children have persistent productive cough, wheeze, hyperexpanded chest deformity and clubbing (Fig. 14.6).

Unusual presentations of CF include sinusitis, nasal polyposis and rectal prolapse.

Investigation

The diagnosis rests on at least two abnormal sweat tests performed by people skilled in the procedure. Localized sweating is induced by iontophoresis with pilocarpine, and sweat is absorbed onto filter paper. In 99% of homozygotes, sweat, sodium and chloride levels are raised over 70 mmol/L.

Mutation analysis is extremely helpful but cannot exclude CF as not all mutations are known. In affected families it forms a reliable test for fetal and neonatal screening.

Pancreatic damage results in raised serum immuno reactive trypsin in the first 6 weeks of life. This can be detected in the blood spots collected for routine neonatal screening. There is a growing consensus that screening of the entire population at birth for CF offers advantage. This remains controversial, but routine screening is performed in some parts of the UK. Available screening tests have high sensitivity but are not specific — this leaves large numbers

of parents worried until they discover that their child does not have CF. Presymptomatic diagnosis, however, allows early introduction of the modern aggressive therapy which has transformed the prognosis.

Treatment and prognosis

The respiratory problems of CF are progressive. Modern aggressive therapy, started at an early age, has transformed the prognosis for CF (Table 14.3). Most children reach adulthood. This is only possible in a multidisciplinary, specialist centre, with medical and auxiliary staff specially trained and familiar with this disease. Gene therapy is an exciting future possibility.

LONG-TERM COMPLICATIONS OF CF

- Respiratory failure
- Psychological/emotional problems
- Diabetes mellitus
- Portal hypertension
- Hepatic cirrhosis
- Cor pulmonale
- Distal intestinal obstruction syndrome
- Male infertility

TREATMENT OF CF

Respiratory	Nutritional	Family
Physiotherapy at least twice every day	Constant monitoring	Education
Early antistaphylococcal prophylaxis	Dietetic supervision	Teach parents/child to do physiotherapy
Aggressive high-dose intravenous antibiotics for exacerbations	High energy/protein 150% of average requirements	Recognition of relapse
Bronchodilators	High fat diet	Home intravenous antibiotics
	Pancreatic enzyme replacement therapy	Genetic counselling
		Financial help (e.g. disability living allowance)
		Emotional support

Table 14.3 Treatment of cystic fibrosis.

OSCE Station: Examination of the respiratory system

Clinical approach:

Check hands
- clubbing
- colour
- perfusion

Check face
- colour
- anaemia
- respiratory distress

Chest

Inspection
Acute signs
- respiratory rate
- recession/increased work of breathing
- added noises (cough, wheeze, etc.)

Chronic signs
- chest shape
- pectus carinatum/AP diameter
- Harrison's sulci

Percussion
- percuss upper, mid and lower zones, anteriorly and posteriorly
- dullness over the heart is normal

Auscultation
- added noises
  ◇ stridor
  ◇ wheeze
  ◇ crackles
  ◇ crepitation
  ◇ rub

James is 14 years old. Please examine his respiratory system

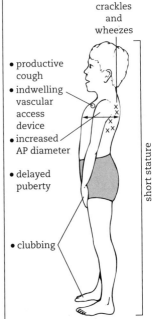

crackles and wheezes

- productive cough
- indwelling vascular access device
- increased AP diameter
- delayed puberty
- clubbing

short stature

James has cystic fibrosis with signs of chronic lung infection and asthma. He has poor growth, and no signs of puberty.

Never forget:

- say hello and introduce yourself
- general health—is the child ill?
- colour—?pale/ ?cyanosis
- quickly assess growth, nutrition and development
- mention the obvious (e.g. drip, leg in plaster)

Look around for:

- inhalers
- sputum pot
- nasogastric tube, gastrostomy
- vascular access device
- oxygen—mask, nasal prongs
- medications

Special points

- evidence of atopic disease (e.g. eczema)
- beware transmitted noises; listen again after asking the child to cough
- percussion is usually unhelpful in children under 2 years, and they don't like it; omit it and explain why
- percuss onto your finger, not direct on-to clavicle
- downward displacement of the liver occurs if the chest is overexpanded

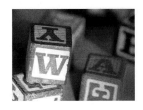

Ear, Nose and Throat

ENT problems are very common in children. The upper respiratory tract is the commonest site of infection in the young child and assessment of the acute illness in children is not complete without examination of the ears, nose and throat (p. 32). Chronic disorders are important causes of long-term morbidity. The early diagnosis of sensorineural and conductive hearing loss is essential if secondary educational and social effects are to be minimized (p. 101). Paediatric specialists in ENT surgery play an essential role in the less frequently seen chronic disorders, such as persistent stridor.

Otitis media

Acute otitis media is common throughout the first 8 years. In the older child the cardinal symptom, earache, makes detection easy; in infants it may not be so obvious. They usually have high fever and are irritable, rolling their heads from side to side, or rubbing their ears. Initially there is mild inflammation of the pars flaccida (the superior part of the tympanic membrane) with dilated vessels running down the handle of the malleus, and an absent light reflex. This progresses to a red, bulging, painful tympanic membrane, perforation and discharge of pus. A mildly pink dull drum may be present in any URTI.

At least half of the incidence of otitis media is viral, but antibiotics are usually given. Pathogens include *Streptococcus pneumoniae* and *Haemophilus influenzae*. Amoxycillin is the antibiotic of choice, and paracetamol is invaluable for the fever and pain.

Mastoiditis, lateral sinus thrombosis, meningitis, and cerebral abscess are rare complications. Persistent aural discharge (chronic suppurative otitis media) is less rare.

Secretory otitis media (glue ear, serous otitis media)

Sticky, serous material accumulates in the middle ear insidiously or after acute otitis media. The symptoms are earache, deafness or a feeling of fullness or popping in the ear. It is especially common in children who have atopy, frequent upper respiratory infections or cleft palate. The eardrum is usually dull and retracted and fluid level may be seen. The malleus handle is more horizontal and appears shorter, broader and whiter. Glue ear is the commonest cause of conductive hearing loss below the age of 10 years (Fig. 15.1). Antibiotics, antihistamines and decongestants may be tried. If there is significant deafness an indwelling tube (*grommet*) is inserted through the eardrum to aerate the middle ear and is left for 6–12 months.

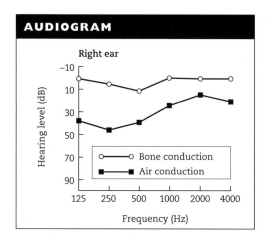

AUDIOGRAM

Fig. 15.1 Audiogram: this child has right, moderate, conductive hearing loss.

Tonsils and adenoids

Lymphoid tissue grows rapidly in the first 5 years of life. Tonsils and adenoids are usually small in infants and reach their greatest relative size between 4 and 7 years. Cervical glands are normally palpable at this age, and readily enlarge in response to local infection.

Acute tonsillitis

This is very common in the age group 2–8 years but uncommon in infants. There is sudden onset of fever, sore throat and dysphagia. Vomiting and abdominal pains are common. The tonsils are enlarged and fiery red; white exudate appears in the tonsillar glands.

Tender cervical lymphadenopathy is usual. Viral and bacterial tonsillitis cannot be distinguished clinically. The commonest bacterial pathogen (30–40%) is beta haemolytic streptococcus. Infectious mononucleosis is associated with nasty tonsillitis in older children.

Paracetamol and cool drinks provide symptomatic relief. Penicillin is often used because it will eradicate streptococci and reduce the risk of complications.

TONSILLITIS: COMPLICATIONS

Complications are rare, but important:

- **Immediate**
  - *Peritonsillar abscess (quinsy):* severe symptoms of tonsillitis and dysphagia. The tonsil appears displaced towards the midline.
  - *Cervical abscess:* marked cervical adenitis is usual at the time of tonsillitis. Occasionally infection localizes in a cervical lymph gland to form an abscess.

- **Delayed**
  - *Acute nephritis* (p. 178) 2–3 weeks after the infection.
  - *Rheumatic fever* (p. 193) 1–2 weeks after the infection.

Obstructive sleep apnoea

In rare cases, enlargement of the tonsils or adenoids tissue causes upper airway obstruction. The leads to difficulty in breathing, which is usually marked by loud snoring and a disturbed abnormal pattern of breathing during sleep. The result of disturbed sleep is tiredness during the day and behavioural problems. In severe cases, poor growth and development and a wide variety of symptoms are seen and occasionally the nocturnal hypoxia may lead to pulmonary hypertension. Recognition is important. Tonsillectomy/adenoidectomy gives good results.

Adenotonsillectomy

INDICATIONS

- Recurrent/persistent tonsillitis (more than 3 attacks a year)
- Obstructive sleep apnoea
- Recurrent otitis media.

Parents seek this operation for a multiplicity of reasons. They need to be told that in general tonsillectomy does not prevent the child catching colds, sore throats or bronchitis: it does not improve the child's appetite or growth.

Sinusitis

The frontal and sphenoidal sinuses do not develop until 5 and 9 years, respectively. The maxillary and ethmoidal sinuses are small in these years and sinusitis is uncommon before the age of 5.

Allergic rhinitis

Recurrent bouts of sneezing, a persistent watery nasal discharge, and watering eyes are typically worse outside in bright sunshine. The nasal mucosa is pale and oedematous. Allergic rhinitis in late spring and early summer in response to grass pollen, is called *hay fever*. Other allergens include dust, animal dander and moulds. A careful history is more likely to identify the allergen than allergy tests. Nose and eye drops are

useful. Therapeutic success with topical cromoglycate or steroids is variable. Some children are helped by antihistamines.

Epistaxis

Nose bleeds usually originate from the anterior inferior corner of the nasal septum (Little's area). Common causes are minor injury and upper respiratory tract infections. Children may alarm everyone by vomiting blood which they have swallowed. First aid consists of sitting the child up and squeezing the nose firmly whilst the child is comforted and told to breathe through the mouth.

Stridor

Stridor is noisy inspiration due to upper airway obstruction, commonly in the larynx. In young children, the larynx is small with walls that are flabby compared with the firm, cartilaginous adult larynx. It is a voice bag, not a voice box, and it collapses and obstructs easily.

Congenital stridor

Stridor caused by abnormalities of the pharynx, larynx or trachea may be audible from birth. The least rare form, 'congenital laryngeal stridor', is due to floppy aryepiglottic folds. It does not cause serious obstruction and gradually disappears as the laryngeal cartilage becomes firmer during the first year of life. If it is severe enough to cause intercostal and suprasternal recession, or if there is no improvement by the age of 3 months, laryngoscopy is advisable.

Acute stridor

In young children, especially infants and toddlers, stridor can progress to serious respiratory obstruction with alarming rapidity.

Hospital admission is therefore mandatory. The main causes of acute stridor are:

1 Acute laryngotracheitis
2 Foreign body in the larnyx (p. 145)
3 Epiglottitis

> In acute stridor with respiratory distress, do not examine the throat: you may precipitate complete airway obstruction.

Acute laryngotracheitis (croup)

This is common, often mild, but sometimes alarming and potentially dangerous. Onset is sudden, often at night, with stridor, harsh cry and a barking cough (croup). If obstruction is marked there may be intercostal and suprasternal recession in addition to stridor.

CROUP

- Age 1–4 years
- Mild/moderate systemic illness
- Viral infection
- Associated URTI
- Intubation rarely needed.

Antibiotics are not needed. Cold humidity gives symptomatic relief. Intravenous fluids may be needed; inhaled steroids may help. In severe cases children should be monitored carefully. Less than 5% of children in hospital require intubation. Nebulized adrenaline provides temporary relief.

Epiglottitis

This child with stridor is acutely ill and feverish. In this serious emergency, the child's airway is in grave danger of complete obstruction: she sits up, drooling because swallowing is difficult. At intubation, the swollen epiglottis may be seen like a cherry. The cause is infection with *Haemophilus influenzae* and septicaemia is common. Prompt antibiotic and supportive treatment are essential. It is prevented by immunization (p. 218).

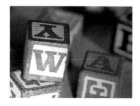

Gastroenterology

Intestinal disorders are usually acute and infective. These are most serious in infancy, when fluid and electrolyte balance can become dangerously disturbed within a matter of hours and cause death or brain damage. Assessment of chronic disorders can be difficult. In most children recurrent abdominal pain, gastro-oesophageal reflux, constipation and persistent diarrhoea are benign and self limiting. Less common but equally important are intestinal obstruction, malabsorption states including coeliac disease and cystic fibrosis. In children, ulcerative colitis and Crohn's disease are uncommon, while peptic ulcers and neoplasm are rare.

Vomiting

Acute-onset vomiting is a common symptom. It is highly-non-specific and a search for non-gastroenterological disease is essential. When vomiting is forceful (projectile), persistent or bile stained, intestinal obstruction or ileus should be considered.

Persistent mild symptoms are very common in babies, who bring up small amounts of food when breaking wind after a feed. This is *possetting*, a normal process, and the baby

- **Feeding errors**
  - Infants: faulty feeding technique
  - Older children: dietary indiscretions

- **Infection**
  - Gastritis (with or without enteritis).
  - Parenteral infections (e.g. tonsillitis, meningitis)
  - Appendicitis

- **Mechanical**
  - Intestinal obstruction, congenital or acquired
  - Gastro-oesophageal reflux

- **Dietary protein intolerance**

- **Raised intracranial pressure**
  - Meningitis, encephalitis
  - Space-occupying lesions (tumour, abscess, haematoma)

- **Psychological problems**
  - Rumination
  - Periodic syndrome (cyclical vomiting)
  - Bulimia

- **Miscellaneous**
  - Travel sickness
  - Poisoning

is happy and gains weight well. Significant vomiting will be accompanied by weight loss, or at least inadequate weight gain.

Gastro-oesophageal reflux

Asymptomatic, infrequent reflux of gastric contents is physiological. Reflux is most common in young infants who effortlessly regurgitate milk over parents, furniture and carpets. The vast majority remain well; reassurance and growth monitoring is all that it justified and symptoms resolve in infancy with maturation of lower oesophageal sphincter function. Sub-optimal weight gain, feeding problems, haematemesis or anaemia and recurrent respiratory symptoms should raise alarm. Investigations include 24 h monitoring of oesophageal pH (in most normal infants acid is found in the oesophagus for less than 6% of the time) and endoscopy.

Reflux is most common and more often severe in infants with cerebral palsy, neurodevelopmental problems, preterm infants, and young children with chronic respiratory disorders. Management includes examination of feeding technique, milk thickeners and antacids. Occasionally, suppression of gastric acid secretion and use of prokinetic agents is indicated.

Haematemesis is not common. Fresh or altered blood may have been swallowed (e.g. epistaxis, tonsillectomy). Acute gastritis and oesophagitis, typically with reflux, oesophageal varices and peptic ulcer should be considered. Exclude bleeding diathesis. If recent haematemesis is suspected check the stools for occult blood.

Diarrhoea and constipation

Diarrhoea or constipation requires detailed enquiry. The number and consistency of stools passed by children, especially infants, is very variable. Breast-fed babies pass loose, bright yellow, odourless stools, between seven times a day and once every

CAUSES OF DIARRHOEA

- **Feeding errors**
  - In infants, too much, too little or the wrong kind
  - In older children, dietary indiscretion

- **Inflammatory lesions**
  - Bacterial or viral infection
  - Post enteritic syndrome
  - Ulcerative colitis/Crohn's disease
  - Giardiasis (lambliasis)
  - Parenteral infections

- **Malabsorption states**
  - Steatorrhoea (e.g. coeliac disease, cystic fibrosis)
  - Disaccharide intolerance

- **Protein losing enteropathy**

- **Food intolerance/allergy**

7 days. Bottle-fed babies pass paler, firmer stools which may cause straining during defaecation. Unless this straining causes pain or rectal bleeding it should not be called constipation. Chronic or severe constipation may lead to abdominal pain, abdominal distension, rectal bleeding, feeding problems and may be associated with emotional and behaviour disorders (p. 123). Chronic constipation in infants or children may lead to faecal impaction and soiling, which may be mistakenly interpreted as diarrhoea.

Many toddlers and some older children continue to have three or four bowel actions a day, after meals. If the stool consistency and weight gain are satisfactory, this is not abnormal. Frequent loose stools are often associated with a rapid transit time, *toddler diarrhoea,* and undigested food may be recognized in the stool within a few hours of being eaten (our personal best was carrots at 20 min).

Abdominal pain

Acute abdominal pain

ABDOMINAL PAIN

Condition	Site of pain and tenderness
Non-organic pain	Central
URTI/tonsillitis	Central/RIF
Pyelonephritis	Loins
Lower lobe pneumonia	Upper abdomen
Mesenteric adenitis	RIF

RIF, right illiac fossa; URTI, upper respiratory tract infection.

This important symptom is highly non-specific. Acute central abdominal pain and vomiting are, for example, common symptoms of tonsillitis. In infants abdominal pain may be inferred from spasms of crying, restlessness and drawing up the knees. From about the age of 2 years, children can indicate the site of a pain. The presence of generalized illness, vomiting, bowel disturbance or fever should prompt detailed appraisal and re-examination after a few hours. Intussusception, complicated hernia and appendicitis are amongst the important surgical causes. Acute abdominal pain is a typical presenting feature in diabetic ketoacidosis (p. 211), Henoch–Schönlein syndrome (p. 176) and sickle cell disease (p. 204).

Appendicitis

Acute appendicitis occurs at all ages but is uncommon under the age of 2 years. The classical history of central abdominal pain, moving to the right ileac fossa, aggravated by movement and associated with fever and acute phase response, raises suspicion which may be confirmed by the finding of localized tenderness in the right iliac fossa. Unfortunately, it is not always that easy. Diagnostic difficulties may be caused by an appendix in an unusual position. Diagnosis of appendicitis is particularly difficult in younger children. The doctor who diagnoses appendicitis before perforation in a 2-year-old deserves praise.

RECURRENT ABDOMINAL PAIN

Features implying organic disease:
- **Pain**
  - Not central
  - Wakes at night
  - Related to food

- **Associated symptoms**
  - Vomiting/diarrhoea
  - Generalized illness
  - Dysuria, daytime enuresis

- **Growth failure**

Chronic abdominal pain

Recurrent symptoms in an otherwise healthy child are common throughout childhood and usually of no serious significance. History, examination, growth assessment and urine microscopy and culture are always justified. The idea that one should exclude all organic causes is naive and usually not possible. In some children, recurrent abdominal pain betrays emotional disorders. In many there is a family history of irritable bowel syndrome or migraine, and the childhood equivalent of irritable bowel syndrome is increasingly well recognized.

Abdominal distension

> The best test for abdominal distension—ask the mother 'Is it distended?'!

Abdominal distension can be difficult to assess because of the great normal variation. Fat babies appear to have bigger tummies than thin, muscular babies. Toddlers are

DEHYDRATION

	Mild	Moderate	Severe
% Bodyweight loss	<5	5–10	>10
Appearance	Normal/ unwell	Anxious/agitated, restless or sleepy	Drowsy/floppy, lethargic
Eyes/fontanelle	Normal	Sunken	Very sunken
Mucous membranes	Normal/dry	Dry	Very dry
Capillary refill	Normal (<2 s)	Normal/prolonged	Prolonged
Peripheral perfusion	Normal	↓ Peripheral perfusion	Cold hands and feet
Blood pressure	Normal	Normal	Low

Table 16.1 Dehydration.

normally rather pot-bellied in comparison with older children and black children in comparison with white.

Dehydration

Early recognition of shock (suboptimal peripheral perfusion) and hypovolaemia is very important in the acutely ill child. The pale, mottled, floppy infant with cold sweaty hands and feet presents an emergency which is readily recognized. No one sign diagnoses dehydration (Table 16.1).

Urine output is reduced as dehydration becomes more severe. Children are very efficient at maintaining central blood pressure in the face of hypovolaemia. Hypotension is a late sign which is not necessary for the diagnosis of moderate dehydration.

Rectal bleeding

Blood in the stools is an alarming symptom, although the cause is often trivial. Bleeding from the duodenum or above will usually cause melaena, although copious bleeding (e.g. swallowed blood after epistaxis or tonsillectomy) may cause red blood to appear with the stool. Blood from the ileum or colon is freely mixed with faecal matter; that from the rectum or anus is only on the surface of the stool. Examination of the perineum, anus and rectal examination (p. 36) may reveal the site of bleeding, or confirm the presence of blood in the stool (Table 16.2).

Piles and rectal carcinoma are very rare in children. Colonoscopy is helpful.

Meckel's diverticulum often contains gastric mucosa which may ulcerate and bleed, causing rectal bleeding and anaemia. Radioactive technetium is selectively taken up by gastric mucosa and this provides the basis for an elegant diagnostic test.

The mouth

The teeth

PREVENTION OF CARIES

- ↓ Plaque-forming organisms
  - Brushing and flossing

- ↓ Carbohydrates
  - Between meals
  - At night

- Adequate fluoride
  - Supplemented drinking water
  - Fluoride toothpaste/tabs

- Regular dental supervision

RECTAL BLEEDING

Site	Condition	Clinical picture
Ileum	Intussusception	Colicky pain; redcurrant jelly stool; palpable mass
	Bleeding, Meckel's diverticulum	Intermittent abdominal pain and bleeding (red or melaena)
Colon	Dysentery (Shigella, Salmonella)	Acute mucoid diarrhoea and pain
	Ulcerative colitis	Chronic mucoid diarrhoea and pain
	Crohn's disease	Abdominal pain, diarrhoea and growth failure
	Intussusception	As above
Rectum	Polyp	Recurrent bleeding: no pain
	Prolapse	Prolapse visible
Anus	Fissure/constipation	On defaecation, much pain and little blood
	Sexual abuse	Dilated/sore anus

Table 16.2 Causes of bleeding per rectum.

There is considerable normal variation in the time of eruption of teeth which may lead to unnecessary worry (p. 27). Preventive dental health is important for all children. Frequent sugary food, especially in early life, should be avoided; we should not forget iatrogenic problems with medicines or vitamin drops. The bottle to suck while falling asleep or the dummy soaked in sweet fluid should be banned. Severe dental problems are more common in children with neurodevelopmental problems and in association with acid reflux.

Include the teeth in the examination of the mouth. It gives an opportunity for congratulation or health education, and occasionally an unexpected alveolar abscess is found to explain a persistent fever or ill health.

Cleft lip and palate

Cleft lip (hare lip) is not usually central but may be unilateral or bilateral. It results from failure of fusion of the maxillary and frontonasal processes. In bilateral cases the premaxilla is anteverted. There is always an associated nasal deformity (p. 60).

Cleft palate may occur alone or with cleft lip. It results from failure of fusion of the palatine processes and the nasal septum. Clefting may cause nasal regurgitation of feeds, and later 'cleft palate speech' because of nasal escape. Otitis media and sensorineural deafness are more common with clefts. Special feeding techniques are often necessary. Submucous cleft palate, in which the muscle of the soft palate is cleft but the overlying mucosa is intact, is much less common.

Early referral to a multidisciplinary team (including orthodontists, plastic surgery, speech therapy) is needed. Most surgical repairs are done within the first 3 months.

Micrognathia and retrognathia

Some babies are born with receding jaws, the jaw being either underdeveloped or displaced backward (Fig. 16.1). In severe cases, the tongue (which is also abnormally far back) obstructs breathing from birth. In combination with cleft palate, this is known as *Pierre–Robin syndrome*. Problems with airway and feeding are most severe in early infancy. In most, mandibular growth and improved coordination lead to resolution.

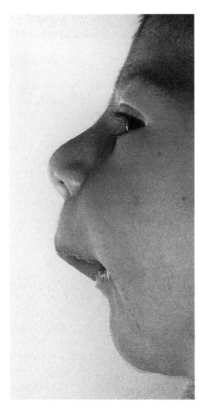

Fig. 16.1 An infant with micrognathia and retrognathia.

Stomatitis

RISK FACTORS FOR CANDIDIASIS

- Extreme prematurity
- Poor hygiene
- Broad-spectrum antibiotics
- Chronic illness
- Malnutrition
- Immunodeficiency
- HIV

Stomatitis due to *Candida albicans* (monilia: thrush) is common in infancy. It appears as tiny white flecks inside the cheeks, on the tongue and on the roof of the mouth. Milk curds are a little similar but are larger and can easily be detached with a spatula. *Candida albicans* will be cultured in large numbers from a swab but can often be cultured from the mouths or throats of healthy children. Treatment includes dealing with risk factors and local application of antifungals (e.g. nystatin, miconazole). It is important to continue local application for a few days after apparent cure, otherwise recurrence is likely. *Candida albicans* may also infect the skin of the napkin area (p. 182).

In older children, stomatitis is usually due to a first infection with herpesvirus hominis Type 1 or coxsackie A virus (p. 224). In *Stevens–Johnson syndrome* severe mouth ulceration is associated with conjunctivitis, erythema multiforme and severe systemic illness.

Hernia

Herniae in children may involve the umbilicus, the diaphragm, the inguinal or femoral regions. They differ in some important ways from hernias in adults.

Umbilical hernia

This is common and harmless. There is a small, well defined, circular defect centred on the umbilicus. Umbilical hernias are always easily reducible and virtually never strangulate. When babies with an umbilical hernia cry the hernia protrudes. Spontaneous cure is usual before the first birthday though it may take up to 5 years. Treatment is reserved for large non-resolving lesions.

Diaphragmatic hernia

This congenital abnormality occurs when one side of the diaphragm is not formed. Abdominal contents herniate into the chest early in fetal life and prevent normal lung growth. Most diaphragmatic hernias are left sided: at birth the abdomen appears scaphoid (empty — literally boat shaped); the apex beat is displaced to the right; pulmonary hypoplasia leads to respiratory failure within hours of birth. A chest X-ray makes the diagnosis clear. Early intubation and positive pressure ventilation are usually necessary to maintain life until surgical repair can be undertaken.

Inguinal hernia

This is common in boys, rare in girls. It is often bilateral. It is very common in extremely preterm infants. A big hernia will form a large swelling in the scrotum, which can be reduced quite easily if the baby is quiet. A small hernia will cause a swelling in the groin which may be visible intermittently. The smaller hernia is more likely to strangulate: be as concerned about the hernia you cannot see as the one you can. Complications are common and spontaneous cure does not occur. Surgical repair should be undertaken at the first convenient moment. The hernial sac is resected and the defect repaired (herniotomy).

Intestinal obstruction

CARDINAL SYMPTOMS

- Vomiting ± bile
- Pain
- Abdominal distension
- Constipation.

The causes of intestinal obstruction vary with age. Gastrointestinal malformation usually presents in the fetus or newborn. In the older infant or child, the single commonest cause is the inguinal hernia. In the younger child, fluid and electrolyte losses rapidly lead to dehydration and circulatory failure.

ESSENTIAL MANAGEMENT

- Early diagnosis
- Correction of fluid and electrolyte losses
- Skilled surgery and anaesthesia.

In the newborn

Fetal swallowing is essential for control of amniotic fluid volume. Obstruction high in the gastrointestinal tract may lead to accumulation of fluid (polyhydramnios). No newborn infant with a history of polyhydramnios should be fed milk without considering intestinal obstruction and ruling out oesophageal atresia (Fig. 16.2).

DEFINITIONS

Atresia: passage not formed
Stenosis: passage narrowed

Oesophageal atresia is usually associated with *tracheo-oesophageal fistula*. There may be polyhydramnios, and shortly after birth the infant is 'bubbly' with oral secretions which cannot be swallowed. Diagnosis must be made before milk is given because fluid cannot reach the stomach and immediate regurgitation will lead to choking, cyanosis and aspiration. This is a disastrous start in life for these infants and they will need urgent surgery. If there is any suspicion of oesophageal atresia, a wide-bore nasogastric tube should be passed to demonstrate patency of the oesophagus. Early diagnosis and skilled surgery offer the best chance of cure. There are other severe defects in about half the cases. Oesophageal and rectal atresia sometimes occur in the same baby.

Atresias at lower levels causes vomiting and distension. In high obstruction, vomiting occurs early. Vomit contains bile if obstruction is below the ampulla of Vater.

OESOPHAGEAL ATRESIA

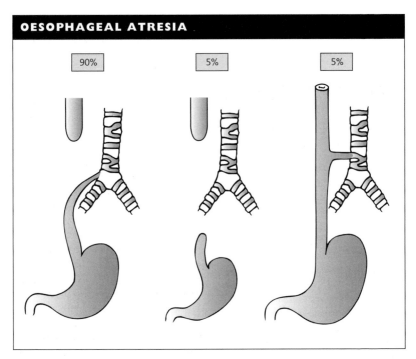

Fig. 16.2 Three forms of oesophageal atresia ± tracheo-oesophageal fistula.

Duodenal atresia and stenosis are particularly common in Down's syndrome. *Rectal atresia* (imperforate anus) is often associated with a rectal fistula to the genitourinary tract. An infant with low, complete obstruction cannot pass meconium, but small quantities may be passed by those with high obstruction.

Other congenital gut abnormalities

Hirschsprung's disease is due to absence of the myenteric plexus in a segment of bowel, most commonly in the rectosigmoid region. Delayed passage of meconium is followed by constipation and distention. Rectal biopsy yields the diagnosis.

Meconium ileus is pathognomonic of cystic fibrosis (p. 150).

In the embryo, the developing gut herniates from the abdominal cavity, returning with a twist so that the caecum ends up in the right iliac fossa. *Malrotation* occurs when this process is incomplete. It may result in obstruction from peritoneal bands compressing the intestine or volvulus.

In *exomphalos* (omphalocele) the normal embryonic herniation development has become permanent. Bowel and other abdominal viscera protrude from the umbilicus, often enclosed in a membrane. *Gastroschisis* describes a serious congenital defect of the abdominal wall with herniation of peritoneal contents. Prior to surgical repair, a nasogastric tube is passed, fluid replacement is given and herniated intestine is wrapped in plastic (cling film).

Infancy and childhood

Intestinal obstruction at later ages may be caused by pyloric stenosis, intussusception, volvulus, strangulated inguinal hernia or other rare causes.

Intussusception

INTUSSUSCEPTION

- Paroxysms of colicky pain
- Between attacks quiet and pale
- Cardinal feature of obstruction
- Redcurrant jelly stool (blood and mucus)
- Sausage-shaped mass (often right upper quadrant).

Intussusception occurs most commonly in infancy. Change in diet and intestinal flora or viral infection causes hypertrophy of Peyer's patches, which may form the apex of the intussusception. Once established, spasms of pain become more frequent and severe. Dehydration and hypovolaemia are common and the intussusception can be felt in the abdomen or occasionally per rectum (Fig. 16.3).

Ultrasound may be helpful in diagnosis. The diagnostic and therapeutic method of choice is air contrast enema. Air is insufflated per rectum and will hopefully reduce the intussusception. Contrast medium can be used in the same way. If reduction is unsuccessful or there is perforation or gangrenous bowel, operation and possibly resection is needed.

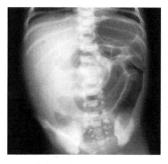

Fig. 16.3 Plain abdominal X-ray showing dilated loops of small bowel.

If air enema is performed within 12 h of intussusception, successful reduction is achieved in over 90%. Diagnostic delay makes surgery more likely.

Pyloric stenosis

Hypertrophic pyloric stenosis occurs in 1 : 150 boys and 1 : 750 girls. Increased incidence in monozygotic twins and close relatives suggests a genetic contribution. It is not congenital (present at birth) and has never been found in stillborn infants. Pathologically, hypertrophy of the circular muscle of the pylorus leads to progressive obstruction (Fig. 16.4).

Symptoms usually begin gradually in the second or third week of life. Vomiting becomes frequent, copious and forceful (projectile vomiting). Weight gain stops and is followed by weight loss. Despite vomiting, he remains ravenous. A test feed is performed to make the diagnosis. Watch the infant feed, a procedure that may take half an hour. As the stomach fills, waves of peristalsis become visible, crossing the epigastrium from left to right. Gastric peristalsis increases until the infant vomits, when the vomitus may shoot out several feet. The hypertrophic pylorus may be felt before the feed begins, but more often at the time of vomiting. It is the shape and size of a large olive and very firm. Diagnosis may be confirmed by ultrasound, demonstrating a large pylorus and a narrow elongated canal. A contrast meal may be necessary for diagnosis.

BLOOD GAS IN PYLORIC STENOSIS

pH 7.50 P_{CO_2} 2.0 kPa Bicarbonate 36 mmol/L
Alkalosis because pH > 7.40; high bicarbonate + low CO_2, therefore: metabolic acidosis

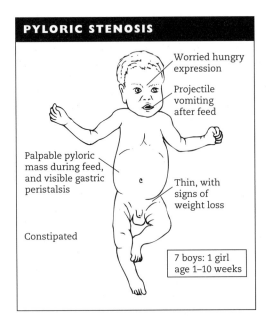

PYLORIC STENOSIS

Worried hungry expression

Projectile vomiting after feed

Palpable pyloric mass during feed, and visible gastric peristalsis

Thin, with signs of weight loss

Constipated

7 boys: 1 girl
age 1–10 weeks

Fig. 16.4 Pyloric stenosis.

Repeated vomiting leads to dehydration and large losses of HCl. The result is a hypochloraemic alkalosis. Successful management demands that the paediatrician corrects electrolyte abnormalities before surgery. In Ramstedt's operation, the pylorus is exposed through a horizontal skin incision and the hypertrophic muscle divided along its length until the mucosa bulges up. Post-operatively most infants will tolerate milk a few hours later and the prognosis is excellent.

Infective diarrhoea

Acute, infective diarrhoea is common. It spreads rapidly through a closed community like a home or a hospital ward. It is potentially lethal, especially in the very young or malnourished. The cause is viral or bacterial, although a similar illness may result from the ingestion of bacterial exotoxins or chemical poisons. Causative organisms may be found in 70%. Rotavirus is found in over 50% of cases and more common bacterial infections include *Campylobacter*, *Salmonella*, *E. coli* and *Shigella*. *Cryptosporidium* is particularly important in immunodeficient children.

 In infants with gastroenteritis:
- Breast feeding should not stop
- Formula milk can be reintroduced as soon as rehydration is achieved.

ORS	
Na	60 (mmol/L)
K	20 (mmol/L)
Cl	60 (mmol/L)
Citrate	10 (mmol/L)
Glucose	90 (mmol/L)

The main danger: diarrhoea and vomiting quickly upset fluid and electrolyte balance. Dehydration must be recognized early (p. 160). The basis of treatment is rehydration and correction of electrolyte balance.

Hypernatraemic dehydration is now rare but remains a dangerous condition. Antibiotics should be reserved for systemic infection. In *Salmonella* and *Shigella* infections, antibiotics may delay clearance of the pathogens. The answer is a beautiful example of applied physiology. The combination of sodium and glucose provides accelerated uptake of salt and water through glucose-coupled sodium cotransport. *Oral rehydration solutions* (ORS) are conveniently made up from prepacked sachets of dry powder. After careful reconstitution, small volumes are given at frequent intervals in order to re-hydrate and then maintain hydration. Only a minority require intravenous rehydration. When hospital admission is needed there must be strict barrier nursing to prevent the spread of infection to others.

> **i** The introduction of ORS has made a major contribution to reduction in worldwide childhood mortality.

Postenteritic syndrome

In less than 5% of gastroenteritis, a combination of lactose intolerance and/or acquired dietary protein intolerance occurs. This results in the return of watery diarrhoea each time milk is reintroduced together with continued weight loss. Careful dietetic appraisal and management usually results in resolution within 2 months.

Malabsorption states

MALABSORPTION

- Abnormal stools
- Poor growth
- Nutrient deficiency

Poor absorption may be specific to one nutrient or generalized. Malabsorption with steatorrhoea is usually due to coeliac disease or cystic fibrosis. Fatty stools are offensive, pale and bulky and frequent. The mother may report difficulty in flushing them down the toilet because of their tendency to float. Abdominal distension due to gas and fluid in the distended bowel, is accompanied by weight loss and muscle wasting.

Coeliac disease

Coeliac disease is the result of sensitivity to the gluten fraction of wheat, rye or other cereals. Symptoms only occur after the introduction of cereals into the diet. Introduction of cereals before the age of 4 months may increase risk of coeliac disease. The classical presentation is now less common. Children present at a later age with a variety of gastrointestinal symptoms, variable growth failure and iron deficient anaemia (Fig. 16.5).

SPECIAL INVESTIGATION OF MALABSORPTION

- Dietary assessment
- Growth assessment
- Stool for fat content and culture
- Clinical/laboratory assessment of nutrition
- Sweat test
- Coeliac disease antibodies
- Jejunal biopsy

The diagnosis of coeliac disease cannot be made without jejunal biopsy, which shows subtotal villous atrophy on histology. It is mandatory to exclude cystic fibrosis and infection with *Giardia lamblia*.

Treatment consists of lifetime exclusion of all foods containing wheat, rye and barley. The response is usually rapid and dramatic over a few weeks, with rapid catch-up growth. Specific nutrient deficits (e.g. iron, fat, soluble vitamins) must be addressed. Regular follow-up of compliance with support from a dietitian is essential.

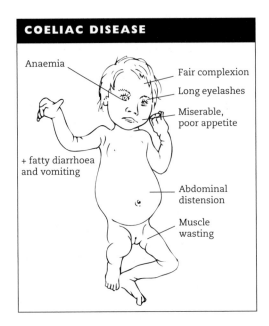

COELIAC DISEASE

Anaemia

Fair complexion

Long eyelashes

Miserable, poor appetite

+ fatty diarrhoea and vomiting

Abdominal distension

Muscle wasting

Fig. 16.5 Classical coeliac disease.

Before committing someone to a life-long gluten-free diet, it is vital to be sure of the diagnosis. Some people with coeliac disease 'tolerate' gluten without acute symptoms, but taking gluten will increase risk of lymphoma. As gluten intolerance in early life is occasionally temporary, it is wise to give a gluten challenge followed by a repeat biopsy at a later date.

Cystic fibrosis

Cystic fibrosis (CF) is the commonest cause of pancreatic malabsorption. Advances in nutritional management have been central to the improvements in the prognosis of CF. CF is dealt with in Chapter 14 (p. 149).

Other gastrointestinal disorders

Food intolerance

Food intolerance is an unwanted abnormal response to food. All studies using double blind challenges have shown that symptoms are too often ascribed to reaction to foods. Food intolerance may be allergic, metabolic (e.g. lactase deficiency), toxic (e.g. food colourings), or irritant (e.g. chilli). Food intolerance including allergy can be secondary to gut disorders (e.g. post-enteritic syndrome and Crohn's disease).

> Commonest food antigens leading to allergy:
> - Cow's milk protein
> - Soya
> - Eggs
> - Wheat
> - Peanut
> - Others: fish, crustacea, nuts, strawberry, additives.

Food allergy is a reproducible clinical reaction to specific foods accompanied by an abnormal immune response. It is commoner in the young and lessens with age, most resolving in infancy and almost all within 3 years of onset. The clinical reaction may be acute and immediate, for instance with anaphylaxis, angioneurotic oedema and urticaria. A more gradual reaction is usual with vomiting, diarrhoea (and even colitis), failure to thrive or eczema.

DIAGNOSIS OF FOOD ALLERGY

Remove antigen ⇒ symptom resolves
Challenge ⇒ symptom recurs

Allergy tests are of limited value in diagnosis, although raised levels of IgE specific to individual food proteins are suggestive of allergy. Skin prick tests are used infrequently. Some believe that food additives (e.g. artificial colourings and flavourings) cause hyperactive behaviour.

An increasing number of infants have acute severe reactions to food antigens. The peanut is the most important of these. The family may need to be trained in resuscitation and some are given adrenaline to use in an emergency. Challenge with food antigen is done for diagnosis and to establish remission. If there is risk of severe reaction, challenges are performed in hospital.

Disaccharide intolerance

Disaccharide intolerance usually involves lactose, and occurs in:
• Post enteritic syndrome (temporary complication of gastroenteritis);
• Coeliac disease or cystic fibrosis (not common);
• Permanent hereditary lactase deficiency (rare).

HYDROLYSIS OF DISACCHARIDES

Lactose ⇒ glucose + galactose
Sucrose ⇒ glucose + fructose

The condition causes a fermentative diarrhoea with frothy explosive stools. A good clinical response to the exclusion of the offending sugar suggests the diagnosis. If the intolerance is temporary lactose may be cautiously reintroduced once recovery from the underlying cause is complete. Formal diagnosis depends on demonstration of disaccharides in the stools, which are acid, a positive hydrogen breath test after ingestion of the suspect sugar, and deficiency of disaccharidases on jejunal biopsy specimens.

Chronic inflammatory bowel disease

INFLAMMATORY BOWEL DISEASE

• Abdominal pain
• Diarrhoea
• Rectal bleeding
• Growth failure

Ulcerative colitis and *Crohn's disease* are not common, although over a quarter of inflammatory bowel disease presents in childhood and Crohn's disease is becoming more common in children. They do not differ in essentials from the adult pattern. Children with the classic symptoms are diagnosed early. Crohn's disease particularly can present with non-specific features, principal amongst these is growth failure and weight loss. Occasionally there may be no gut symptoms. Specific clues to Crohn's disease include oral disease and perianal sepsis, fissures and skin tags.

An acute phase response is found on investigation. Contrast studies and isotope label white cell scans are helpful. The diagnosis rests on histology of biopsy specimens obtained at endoscopy.

Treatment is empirical and not very satisfactory. Remission may be induced by steroids and maintained with salicylate derivatives. Crohn's disease may be managed with elemental diet; other immunosuppressive agents are helpful. Surgery is usually avoided in childhood. Colitis in infants is usually due to cow's milk intolerance and responds to the exclusion of cow's milk.

Hepatic failure

Hepatocellular failure is rare. It may occur in fulminating viral infections (e.g. hepatitis, Epstein–Barr [p. 223]), severe obstructive jaundice, metabolic disorders (p. 215) and a variety of different poisons including paracetamol. Early referral to a specialist centre for investigation and consideration for liver transplant is essential.

Reye's syndrome is the name given to a devastating illness of young children in which there is an acute encephalitis together with acute liver failure. There is a high mortality and at autopsy the children have fatty degeneration of the liver, kidneys and heart. The cause is unknown but because of a possible association with therapeutic doses of salicylate, aspirin should not be used as an analgesic or antipyretic in children under 12 years.

Helicobacter pylori

The discovery of this organism has revolutionized the treatment of peptic ulceration in adults. Its association with peptic ulcers, which are rare in children, is strong. Colonization appears to occur in childhood. Diagnosis may be made by serology, a stable isotope test which exploits helicobacter's ability to split urea and produce carbon dioxide, and endoscopic biopsy. If helicobacter is found, most prescribe eradication therapy.

Giardiasis and worms

Giardia lamblia is a protozoon which commonly inhabits the gut canals in children without disturbing their health. Occasionally it causes chronic diarrhoea with semi formed, light-coloured stools and may lead to malabsorption. Cysts are be identified in the stools, but their presence does not establish that they are causing disease. Isolation of organisms from duodenal aspirate is more significant. Treatment is with metronidazole.

Threadworms (*Enterobius vermicularis*) are relatively common. They cause no symptoms apart from peri-anal itching which may disturb sleep. Diagnosis is made by seeing the worms on the perianal skin or stool, or by demonstrating ova from the peri-anal region, best achieved by the use of cellophane swabs or Sellotape. Mebendazole is the drug of choice for children over 2 years. Apparent failure is usually due to re-infection. Success is then often achieved by treating the whole family, including parents.

The *roundworm* (*Ascaris lumbricoides*) is uncommon in Europe. There are usually no symptoms before a worm is passed with the stools. *Tapeworms* (*Taenia saginata* and *T. solium*) present with the passage of segments. Treatment may be difficult. *Hookworm* (*Ancylostoma*) is an important cause of iron deficient anaemia in developing countries.

OSCE Station: Examination of the abdomen

Clinical approach:

Check hands
- clubbing
- colour
- perfusion

Check face
- colour
- anaemia
- jaundice

Abdomen

Inspection
- distension/swelling
- movement with breathing
- scars/previous surgery
- prominent blood vessels

Percussion
- demonstrate shifting dullness/fluid thrill
- to assess size of liver

Auscultation
- normal, absent or increased bowel sounds

Palpation
- gentle palpation
- tenderness—watch closely and ask if it hurts
- assess size and identify
  ◦ liver
  ◦ spleen
  ◦ kidneys
- describe masses
  ◦ consistency
  ◦ movement
  ◦ tenderness
- genitalia (inspect/ ?descended testes)
- herniae

Please examine Abdul's abdomen. He is 10 years old

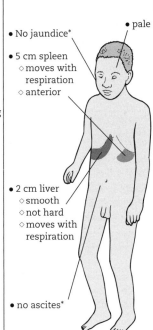

- No jaundice*
- pale
- 5 cm spleen
  ◦ moves with respiration
  ◦ anterior
- 2 cm liver
  ◦ smooth
  ◦ not hard
  ◦ moves with respiration

- no ascites*

- no clubbing*
- generally well
- good nutrition*

(* no signs of chronic liver disease —important negatives)

Abdul has β thalassaemia.

Never forget:

- say hello and introduce yourself
- general health—is the child ill?
- colour—?pale/ ?jaundice
- quickly assess growth, nutrition and development
- mention the obvious (e.g. drip, leg in plaster)

Look around for:

- oral/dental disease
- nasogastric tube/ gastrostomy
- special formula feeds
- nutritional supplements

Special points

- never do a rectal examination in an OSCE
- examination of the genitalia or perianal area should not be done if a child is old enough to be embarrassed by it
- scars from renal surgery may be posterior
- learn techniques for examination of liver, spleen and kidneys
- liver is palpable in healthy infants, and spleen in some healthy newborns

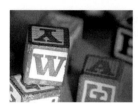

Bones and Joints

Structural variation and congenital abnormalities

The normal flat-footed baby becomes a bow-legged toddler and then a knock-kneed primary schoolchild before growing into a graceful adolescent. One has to decide whether the source of the parents' concern is normal variation or something requiring investigation and treatment (Fig. 17.1).

The child should be examined standing and lying in order to detect abnormality of posture, and to check for equal size and length of the limbs. The child should be observed walking or running, and the shoes examined for abnormal wear.

Flat feet

At birth the feet look flat. When children start to stand, at the end of the first year, the feet still look flat because there is a large pad of fat on the soles. The child starts to walk on a wide base with the feet everted and the tibiae externally rotated and the feet still look flat. By the 3rd year the eversion and external rotation have diminished and the feet begin to appear to have a normal plantar arch.

Bow legs (genu varum)

Bow legs are commonest from 0 to 2 years.

The knees may be 5 cm apart when the feet are together: the toes point medially. If the degree of bowing is gross, rickets should be excluded (p. 81).

Knock knees (genu valgum)

This is most apparent at 3–4 years of age. When the knees are together, the medial tibial malleoli may be up to 5 cm apart. In obese children the separation may be even greater but by the age of 12, the legs should be straight. Separation of over 10 cm or unilateral knock knee requires an X-ray and, probably, a specialist opinion.

Scoliosis

A lateral curve of the spine is commonly seen in babies and may be associated with skull asymmetry. Generally it is a postural scoliosis which goes when the baby is suspended and which has completely gone by the age of 2 years. Scoliosis is again common at adolescence, especially in girls. If the scoliosis disappears on bending forward, it is postural and will resolve; whereas a hump on flexion is abnormal (Fig. 17.2). Asymmetry of scapulae, shoulders or chest configuration may be more conspicuous than the spinal curve. If scoliosis is not postural, orthopaedic referral is important.

Scoliosis may be associated with vertebral anomalies (spina bifida,

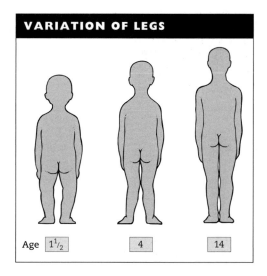

Fig. 17.1 Normal variation of legs with age.

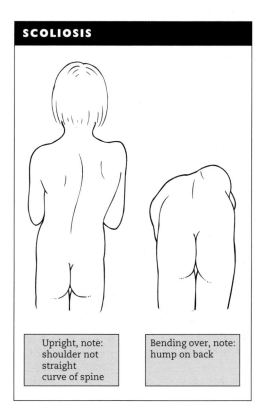

Fig. 17.2 Structural scoliosis becomes more obvious when she bends to touch her toes.

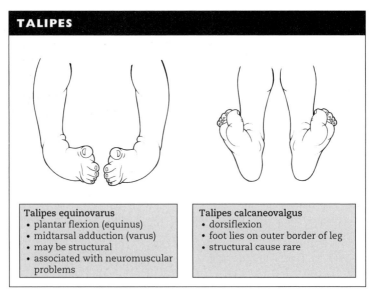

TALIPES

Talipes equinovarus
- plantar flexion (equinus)
- midtarsal adduction (varus)
- may be structural
- associated with neuromuscular problems

Talipes calcaneovalgus
- dorsiflexion
- foot lies on outer border of leg
- structural cause rare

Fig. 17.3 Two forms of talipes.

hemivertebrae) or muscle weakness or imbalance (muscular dystrophy, cerebral palsy), but is idiopathic in 95% of cases.

Talipes (club foot)

Minor degrees of talipes are common at birth, resulting from mechanical pressure *in utero*. If the foot with talipes equinovarus can be fully dorsiflexed and everted so that the little toe touches the outside of the leg without undue force, it can be expected to correct itself with time. If it cannot be so overcorrected, splintage or surgery is needed. The sooner treatment is begun the better the outcome. Usually talipes calcaneovalgus is easily corrected by simple exercises (Fig. 17.3).

Congenital neuromuscular problems and defects of the spinal cord such as spina bifida are commonly associated with severe talipes.

Congenital dislocation of the hip (CDH)

RISK FACTORS FOR CDH

- Breech
- Positive family history
- Girls > boys
- Any other neuromuscular or joint problem (e.g. spina bifida, talipes equinovarus)

Dislocated hips are associated with joint laxity and acetabular dysplasia. Postural factors play a role in their causation.

Diagnosis is made by specifically testing the hips (OSCE, p. 180).

All babies should be examined in the neonatal period and at intervals during the first year. X-ray examination is unreliable in the first month; ultrasound is more reliable and may be used for screening all babies.

One in 60 babies is found to have hip instability at birth: 85% recover spontaneously, but the remainder persist. Early splinting is successful within 2 months in most neonates. If undetected in the neonatal period, it may not become apparent until the parents worry about their 2-year-old's limp. At that age treatment is more traumatic and less successful.

> **i** Screening tests for dislocated hips are not 100% sensitive (cases are missed) or 100% specific (the test may be abnormal in a normal infant).

Osteogenesis imperfecta

This is a group of rare genetic conditions due to mutations in the genes encoding for collagen. They are characterized by brittle bones and lax ligaments. In the lethal forms (dominant mutations or recessive inheritance) multiple fractures occur *in utero*. In less severe cases (usually dominant inheritance) children may merely be prone to fractures. Affected children may have blue sclerae and develop deafness in adult life.

Skeletal dysplasia

There are a large number of generalized congenital skeletal dysplasias which are rare. Many are genetically determined. The best known is *achondroplasia* (the circus dwarf), due to an autosomal dominant gene. In 50% a new mutation occurs, both parents being normal. There is extreme short stature with disproportionate shortness of limbs, and a large skull vault because of the small skull base. Intelligence is normal.

Several other varieties of short-limbed dwarfism are incompatible with survival after birth. Accurate diagnosis is important for genetic counselling.

Osteomyelitis (osteitis)

Pyogenic infection of bone is commoner in children than adults, and in boys than girls.

The usual site is the metaphysis of one of the long bones, particularly in the legs. At all ages except infancy, *Staphylococcus pyogenes* is the commonest pathogen. The sources of infection and portal of entry are uncertain.

OSTEOMYELITIS

Symptoms
- Fever
- Variable pain, illness
- Pseudoparesis
- Localized, acute tenderness
- Redness, swelling

Investigations
- Blood count ?neutrophilia
- C-reactive protein↑
- Blood culture
- Radio-isotope scan
- X-rays

The severity of symptoms varies greatly. An infant may merely refuse to use the affected limb (pseudoparesis).

X-ray is normal at first: after 2 or more weeks rarefaction and periosteal new bone formation may be seen. Radioisotope bone scan is usually abnormal from the start. Osteomyelitis is a most serious condition. Future bone growth is in jeopardy. Intensive treatment in hospital is needed. Large doses of antibiotic that is effective against penicillin resistant staphylococci are given (e.g. flucloxacillin).

If treatment is given early, complete resolution occurs in most cases. If diagnosis is delayed surgical drainage is more likely to be needed.

Arthritis

Arthritis is characterized by a painful inflamed joint in which there is limitation of movement in all directions (Table 17.1). There may be swelling due to fluid in the joint, and redness and heat of the overlying

CAUSES OF ARTHRITIS

Those that may result in permanent joint damage
Juvenile chronic arthritis
Acute suppurative arthritis due to blood-borne infection. This is treated with
  aspiration, antibiotics and splintage
Haemarthrosis (bleeding into joints) in children with coagulation disorders mimics
  acute arthritis

Those that usually resolve completely (synovitis)
Trauma, especially in schoolchildren
Reactive arthritis, secondary to viral infections, e.g., rubella (and immunization)
  mumps and chickenpox
Henoch–Schönlein syndrome
Serum sickness and generalized allergic reactions
Rheumatic fever

Table 17.1 Causes of arthritis.

skin. The joint itself is usually painful. Pain arising in the hip may be referred to the knee.

Juvenile chronic arthritis

Defined as a chronic arthritis developing before the age of 16 and persisting for more than three months, with other primary diseases excluded. It is much less common than in adults. The rare systemic form *(Still's disease)* usually presents about the age of 3 or 4; other forms may occur at any age (Table 17.2).

Young children may present with systemic illness—swinging fever, splenomegaly, lymphadenopathy, erythematous rash—and little or no joint involvement initially. The high ESR and polymorph leucocytosis may suggest infection, and tests for rheumatoid and antinuclear factors are negative.

Older children present with one or more painful, swollen joints and little or no systemic upset. Knees, hips, wrists, ankles and elbows are commonly involved. Neighbouring muscles waste quickly. The term *juvenile rheumatoid arthritis* is used when the small joints of the hands and feet, the cervical spine and the temporomandibular joints are involved and tests for rheumatoid

factor are positive. In juvenile *ankylosing spondylitis*, the knees and hips are often involved before the spine and sacro-iliac joints, and the children (mostly boys) are usually HLA type B27.

At least 50% of children make a complete recovery, but in others the disease is progressive and crippling. Iridocyclitis is an important complication. Physiotherapy, splintage and the rational use of drugs form the basis of treatment. Non-steroidal anti-inflammatory drugs are appropriate for cases of mild to moderate severity. Systemic steroids are often necessary. Methotrexate and anti-cytokine antibodies are used in severe cases.

Other collagen diseases

Systemic lupus erythematosus (SLE), polyarteritis nodosa, dermatomyositis and the other collagen disorders are rare in children. SLE tends to occur in adolescent girls, particularly black races. It tends to present as a multisystem disorder: many of the manifestations subside during treatment with corticosteroids.

Henoch–Schönlein syndrome (anaphylactoid purpura)

The syndrome is commonest in children

JUVENILE ARTHRITIS

	Joints involved	Systemic illness
65% Pauciarticular	Up to four large joints: hip, knee, ankle	Negligible, but uveitis in ANA + and young onset
20% Systemic (Still's disease)	Arthalgia/myalgia later joint involvement	Spiking fever, rash, pains, anaemia, hepato-splenomegaly
15% Polyarticular	More than four symmetrical	Negligible

ANA, antinuclear antibody.

Table 17.2 Juvenile chronic arthritis.

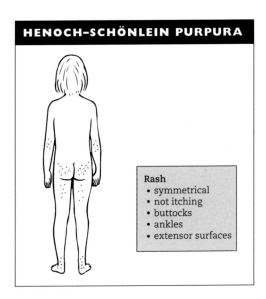

Rash
- symmetrical
- not itching
- buttocks
- ankles
- extensor surfaces

Fig. 17.4 Henoch–Schönlein purpura.

aged 2–10 and is made up of a pathogno-monic purpuric rash and involvement of one or more of the following: joints, alimentary system and kidneys (Fig. 17.4).

Skin
The rash is distributed over extensor surfaces of the limbs, particularly about the ankles and on the buttocks. It begins as a maculopapular, or urticarial, red rash, which gradually becomes purpuric (resulting from the vasculitis, the platelet count is normal). Swelling of the face, hands and feet is common and subcutaneous bleeds may occur.

Joints
Pain (arthralgia) of medium-sized joints is common and may progress to an obvious arthritis with red, swollen, tender joints.

Alimentary system
Colicky abdominal pain occurs and may be severe enough to mimic an acute abdominal emergency. Vomiting and diarrhoea are common, haematemesis and melaena less

common, and intussusception or perforation very rare.

Kidneys

Haematuria and proteinuria are common. With more severe involvement, the glomerulonephritis causes an acute nephritic syndrome, a nephrotic syndrome or renal insufficiency. The renal complications are responsible for the main morbidity and mortality of Henoch–Schönlein syndrome.

The various groups of symptoms generally present within a week of each other, but may occur in any order and persist for several weeks. Recurrence may occur for several months after onset. The cause is unknown and treatment is symptomatic.

Rheumatic fever

Rheumatic fever is still an important cause of acquired heart disease in children throughout the world, but in Europe it has become rare. It results from a sensitivity reaction to a group A beta-haemolytic streptococcal infection. Typically there has been acute tonsillitis 1–4 weeks previously.

Arthritis 'flits' between the medium-sized joints from day to day. Cardiac involvement may lead to scarred valves, typically mitral stenosis and aortic incompetence. The rare serpiginous red rash (erythema marginatum) is pathognomonic. The commoner erythema nodosum is less specific. Serial antistreptolysin O (ASO) titres are elevated. Treatment includes anti-inflammatory agents and penicillin prophylaxis against recurrence.

Osteochondritis and epiphysitis

These terms are applied to bone changes that occur, particularly in epiphyses of children, as a result of avascular necrosis.

They present as bone pain, with local swelling and tenderness. There is limitation of movement and adjacent muscle wasting. Those that occur in weight-bearing joints are the most important, as permanent damage may occur. The best example is *Perthes' disease* which affects the femoral head of children (usually boys) aged 5–8 years. It causes a limp and pain (which may

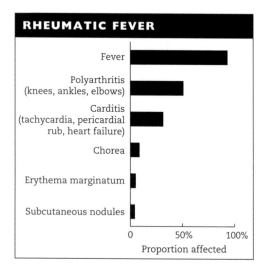

Fig. 17.5 Rheumatic fever signs.

be referred to the knee). The femoral head is softened and will become misshapen if weight-bearing continues, leading to osteoarthritis in early adult life. Treatment with non-weight-bearing calipers allows a reasonably active life until the condition resolves, which may take 2–3 years.

If the affected bone is not a weight-bearing one, the consequences are minimal. Children aged 10–15 are particularly prone to develop transient inflammation of the tuberosity of the tibia (*Osgood–Schlatter disease*). This usually resolves satisfactorily without treatment.

OSCE Station: Testing for dislocation of the hips

Clinical approach:

Inspection
- difference in leg length
- skin creases or asymmetry
- associated abnormalities

ABduct both hips
- they should ABduct fully
- there should be symmetry

Ortolani's sign
- the femoral head clunks back into the acetabulum at 45–60 degrees of ABduction

Barlow's manoeuvre
- support the pelvis on a firm surface or your hand
- flex and ADduct the hip
- apply posterior and lateral pressure to attempt to dislocate the hip
- ABduct the hip, and see if the hip relocates

This model is used for teaching examination of the hips in the newborn. Please show me how this examination is done

ABduction

Ortolani's test: both hips are ABducted fully until they lie flat on the bed. A dislocated hip will not ABduct.

Barlow's manoeuvre

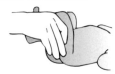

examiner's right hand holding thigh, with finger on greater tronchanter

examiner's left hand supporting pelvis

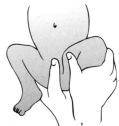

maintaining pressure the hip is ABducted

if right hip is dislocatable, the hip will 'clunk' back into place during ABduction.

In the exam, a teaching model with an abnormal hip is likely to be used

Never forget:

- say hello and introduce yourself
- general inspection— has the infant any congenital abnormality?
- quickly assess general health
- mention the obvious (e.g. drip, leg in plaster)

Look around for:

- hip splints—devices designed to hold the hips in ABduction
- hip harness–similar device with straps that go over the shoulder
- double nappies

Special points

- ligamentous clicks (like you get in your fingers) are of dubious significance
- describe tests as normal or abnormal —it is much more clear than positive/ negative
- Barlow's is easier if you support the pelvis with one hand and test one hip at a time
- make sure someone takes you through these specialized techniques

CHAPTER 18

Skin

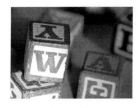

Skin disorders are common in children. The infant's skin with its thin epidermis and immature glands is particularly liable to infection and blistering. Birthmarks, rashes and eczema are common in pre-school children. The incidence of skin disease declines until adolescence when acne is common.

Birthmarks

Birthmarks may involve blood vessels (naevus, haemangioma) or an excess of pigment in the skin. Despite their name, haemangiomata are malformations of blood vessels, not neoplasms. The main types of naevi are:

Stork mark (salmon patch)

This is a flat, pinkish capillary haemangioma on the nape of the neck, the eyelids and between the eyebrows. It fades gradually over the first 2 years (Fig. 18.1).

Strawberry mark

This is a soft, raised, bright red capillary haemangioma (Fig . 18.2). Sometimes it involves deeper tissues and is combined with cavernous haemangioma which gives it a blue tinge. Common sites are the head, neck and trunk. It is not apparent until a few days after birth, and usually enlarges during the first 6 months. Thereafter sunken whitish areas develop in the lump and it gradually becomes paler and flatter. Most have disappeared by the age of 7 years. Treatment is best reserved for the very few that are extremely unsightly, do not regress spontaneously, or are expanding rapidly. In general spontaneous regression does not leave a noticeable scar, whilst treatment often does.

Port wine stain (naevus flammeus)

Port wine stain is a capillary haemangioma (Fig. 18.1). Since it is flat and, in early life, pale pink it is easily overlooked in the infant, but it darkens to form a flat purple patch of skin which looks ugly. It does not fade. Treatment is difficult. Good results have been achieved using laser, but camouflage with cosmetics is often the best treatment. *Sturge–Weber syndrome* is a rare association of a unilateral port wine stain of the face (including the areas supplied by the divisions of the trigeminal nerve) and an intracranial haemangioma of the pia-arachnoid on the same side. Affected children may present with seizures, hemiplegia, learning problems or glaucoma.

Abnormal pigmentation

Moles usually develop after the age of 2. They are common and rarely cause anxiety. Single café-au-lait spots are without significance, but five or more patches greater than 0.5 cm in diameter suggest *neurofibro-*

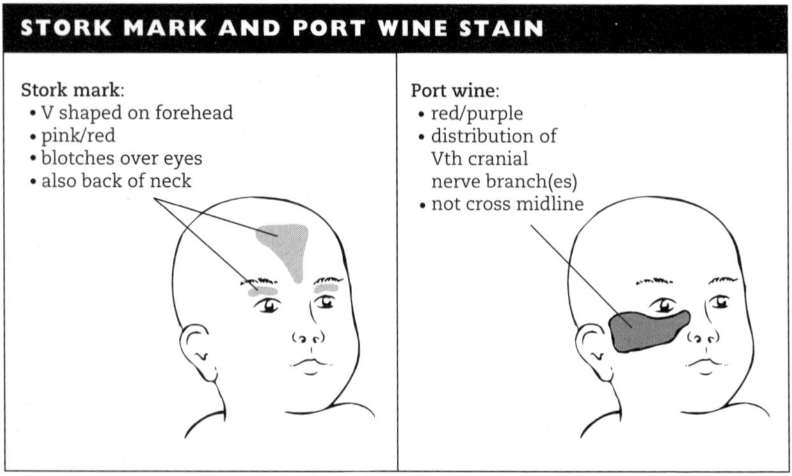

STORK MARK AND PORT WINE STAIN

Stork mark:
- V shaped on forehead
- pink/red
- blotches over eyes
- also back of neck

Port wine:
- red/purple
- distribution of Vth cranial nerve branch(es)
- not cross midline

Fig. 18.1 Stork mark and port wine stain.

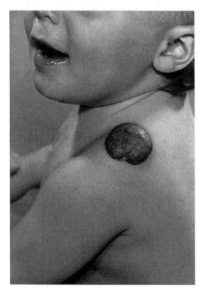

Fig. 18.2 Strawberry naevus.

matosis. Pigmented and de-pigmented lesions are seen in *tuberose sclerosis.*

Albinism

Albinism consists of a group of genetically determined metabolic disorders characterized by deficient pigmentation. In white people autosomal recessive varieties affect the skin, hair and often the eyes. In black people dominant, partial albinism is more common and does not affect the eyes.

Mongolian blue spots

These are large blue-grey patches, most common over the lumbosacral area and buttocks, and may be mistaken for bruises. They are very common in infants of oriental, Asian or negro stock, but rare in white children. They gradually fade and are rarely visible at the age of 10.

Rashes

Napkin rash

Eruptions of the napkin area are common in infants. Characteristically, an erythematous rash affects the convexities of the buttocks, inner thighs and genitalia. The skin creases, which do not come into contact with the nappy, are spared. At its simplest it may merely be an irritant rash caused by wet nappies. Fresh urine does not injure the skin, but prolonged contact with stale urine which has broken down to form ammonia products does (*ammoniacal dermatitis*). In severe cases, papules and vesicles form which ulcerate, leaving a moist surface which easily becomes secondarily infected with either pyogenic organisms or *Candida*. Secondary infection with candida usually involves the skin creases. It causes a moist erythematous rash with oval macules and vesicles, a pimply margin and scattered satellite papules.

Nappy rashes are not confined to babies who have poor care. Some babies have a more sensitive skin than others, and are prone to develop the rash. This must be explained to the mother to dispel needless guilt. However, grossly ulcerated and chronic napkin rashes are a sign of bad care, including infrequent changing.

Treatment is based on frequent and prompt changing of wet nappies including washing and drying the baby's perineum carefully: rubbing a barrier cream or benzalkonium cream on the napkin area. In severe cases the most effective treatment is exposure of the moist rash in a warm dry environment, leaving the nappies off for a few days, together with the use of a steroid cream to suppress the inflammation. Secondary infection requires local bactericidal or fungicidal cream.

Cradle cap (seborrhoea)

Cradle cap is as common in infants as dandruff is in older children. It is a thick, light brown crust over the top of the scalp which may look quite difficult to remove. Most pharmacists sell proprietary brands of medicated shampoo or baby oil with which to wash the baby's scalp. Regular washing of the scalp helps to prevent recurrence.

Some babies develop a more generalized inflammatory skin reaction (*seborrhoeic dermatitis*) particularly affecting the groins,

axillae and neck. Although the skin may be very red and macerated with greasy scaling, it is not irritant and usually resolves within a few weeks. Secondary infection with bacteria or candida may occur.

Eczema

A similar but more troublesome rash is often the first sign of *infantile eczema*. This may be restricted to two or three small lesions or may involve virtually the whole skin surface. Skin cracks behind the pinnae are almost pathognomonic of infantile eczema. The rash is erythematous, scaly or weeping and intensely itchy. Scratching frequently leads to secondary infection. The condition fluctuates, resolves completely in half the children by the age of 2, but in others persists in a mild form or periodically recurs. After infancy *flexural eczema* is seen. Prolonged inflammation leads to thick lichenified skin and local lymph gland enlargement. The condition tends to improve, and becomes more manageable as the child becomes older (Fig. 18.3).

ECZEMA TREATMENTS

- Emollient creams/ointments
- Bath oil, aqueous emollient
- Topical steroids or tar paste
- Bactericidal creams
- Antihistamines for itching
- Night gloves/mittens to limit scratching
- Occlusive dressings

Environmental factors, including food intolerance, should be considered and for children with severe eczema an exclusion diet is worthy of trial. The child with eczema should avoid contact (particularly kissing) with someone who has herpes simplex (cold sore) because of the risk of developing widespread *eczema herpeticum*.

Eczema is common in atopic children whose families give a history of asthma, eczema, urticaria or hay fever: the child is also at risk for asthma and hay fever.

> **i** Atopic eczema affects 3% of pre-school children

Psoriasis

Onset of this unsightly skin condition is commonly seen at the age of 10–11 and in the early 40s. It is genetically determined and at all ages stress seems to be a provocative factor. The typical lesions are silvery scales on top of a circumscribed salmon-red base. Most types affect principally the extensor surface of the limbs and the scalp; they do not itch. Coal tar ointment and shampoo is the treatment of choice. *Guttate psoriasis*, found mainly on the trunk, appears 2–3 weeks after a streptococcal infection such as tonsillitis.

Impetigo

This skin infection is usually due to *Staphylococcus aureus* though it is often complicated by streptococcus. It commonly involves the face, around the mouth and nose, and the hands. It begins as a flaccid blister which rapidly ulcerates producing exudate that dries in a golden brown crust over the red itching skin beneath. Spread may be rapid and scratching may spread it to other parts of the body or to other members of the family. It is very contagious, so the child should be excluded from school until it is healed. Impetigo frequently complicates ezcema, papular urticaria, herpes simplex, scabies or pediculosis.

The lesions respond rapidly to bathing with cetrimide and water to remove the crusts, followed by antibiotic ointment and, if necessary, a course of oral antibiotic. The family must be warned about the risk of becoming infected themselves and the affected child should use a separate towel and face cloth.

Urticaria (hives, nettle rash)

Urticaria is common in children, especially under the age of 5. It is characterized by red

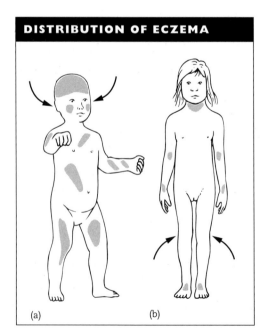

DISTRIBUTION OF ECZEMA

(a)   (b)

Fig. 18.3 Distribution of eczema: (a) in infancy: cheeks, scalp, behind the ears and may be generalized: (b) in later childhood: skin flexures are affected, particularly antecubital and popliteal fossae.

blotches and whitish weals that itch, and disappear and reappear over a period of hours or days. Sometimes sensitivity to a particular drug or food appears to be responsible.

Oral antihistamines are effective; adrenaline injection is reserved for severe anaphylactic episodes involving angio-oedema of the face and mouth.

Papular urticaria consists of hard papules most often on the limbs. They appear in crops and itch so that secondary infection is common. In many children, they are associated with insect bites, fleas (including from pets), lice and bed bugs. Papular urticaria tends to recur for a few years each summer.

Erythema nodosum

The shiny red lumps are 1–3 cm in diameter and may be extremely tender. They are most commonly distributed symmetrically over the front of the shins, but do occur elsewhere. During the first week they become more protuberant, purple and painful, then during the next 2 weeks gradually subside and look like old bruises. They may occur at intervals in crops. Although they are thought to represent a hypersensitivity phenomenon to certain stimuli, the

---

ERYTHEMA NODOSUM — CAUSES

- Streptococcal infection

- Primary tuberculosis

- Drug reaction

- Diseases
  - Inflammatory bowel disease
  - Lupus erythematosus
  - Sarcoidosis

- Idiopathic

---

provocative stimulus frequently cannot be identified.

Warts

Warts are most common in childhood, probably because of the opportunity for contact spread of the responsible virus. The average life of a wart is 9 months, so treatment is usually reserved for long-lasting warts. The variety of available treatments and magic cures is a fair indication of the therapeutic problem and the variable natural history. Topical keratolytics and cryotherapy can be used.

Warts are usually painless; however, a plantar wart (*verruca*) is often painful because the overlying hard skin presses into the foot on walking. Children with plantar warts should be allowed to use swimming baths, but should be advised to cover the wart with a waterproof plaster to lessen the chance of transmission.

Infestations

Pediculosis

The commonest louse infestation in childhood is with the head louse (*Pediculosis capitis*). The insects live close to the scalp and feed on blood which they obtain with their sucking mouth parts. It causes irritation, and the combination of the bites and frequent scratching leads to impetigo and enlarged occipital and cervical lymph glands. The bites may resemble purpura confined to the neck and shoulders. Sometimes the lice can be seen, but more often just the tiny whitish eggs (*nits*) are seen attached singly to the hair. They can be identified with certainty beneath a microscope: they are ovoid with one blunt end and one pointed end by which they are stuck to the hair shaft. Regular use of a fine toothed 'nit comb' will remove eggs from the hair. If necessary, anti-lice shampoo or scalp lotion is used by the whole family. Other members of the home should be examined for similar infestations.

> Head lice are commonest at the age of 6–9 years and occur in all social classes.

Scabies

The mite *Sarcoptes scabiei* lays its eggs in burrows beneath the skin. The larva migrates and burrows into the skin, gradually developing into the adult mite, which re-emerges, becomes impregnated and burrows to lay more eggs. After 2–6 weeks the child becomes sensitized and develops a very itchy papulovesicular rash. In older children, this is most marked in the inter-digital spaces, wrist flexures and anterior axillary folds. In infants, it frequently involves the face, trunk and feet.

The burrows can be seen as small, linear elevations of skin adjacent to a small vesicle, but they are often obscured by excoriation and secondary infection. Scabies should be considered as a possible cause for any unexplained itching rash, and strongly suspected if another family member is affected. Definitive diagnosis may be made by microscopic identification of a mite from one of the burrows. The infestation is transferred by bodily contact, so that other members of the family are usually affected, and all those living together should be treated at the same time. One or two applications of malathion or permethrin are required and disinfestation of clothing and bedding is advised.

OSCE Station: Examination of the skin

Clinical approach:

- careful inspection
- ask child if the rash itches or hurts
- if infection, look for local lymph nodes

Inspection
- colour—is it red?
- distribution/symmetry
- evidence of itching
- added infection

Palpation
- does is blanch?
- is it raised—palpable?
- local lymph nodes

You should recognize:

- common birthmarks
  ◇ haemangiomas
  ◇ strawberry naevus
  ◇ port wine mark
  ◇ stork mark
- eczema (distribution with age/excoriation)
- nappy rashes
- common pigmentation problems
  ◇ mongolian blue spots
  ◇ albinism
- purpura
- impetigo
- psoriasis

Lizzie is 20 months old. She has a skin rash. Please describe the rash

- generally dry skin, with areas of erythematous, scaly rash

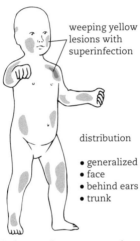

weeping yellow lesions with superinfection

distribution

- generalized
- face
- behind ears
- trunk

Lizzie scratches as you watch

- she has a wheezy cough, and runny nose

Lizzie has eczema (atopic dermatitis).

Never forget:

- say hello and introduce yourself
- general health—is the child ill?
- colour—?pale/ ?cyanosed
- quickly assess growth, nutrition

Look around for:

- skin creams
- occlusive bandaging
- nail changes
- associated systemic disease (e.g. asthma in atopy)

Special points

- avoid describing all rashes as maculo-papular!
- if you are confident it is psoriasis, say it is and give your reasons
- chicken pox and infectious rashes are unlikely in the examination

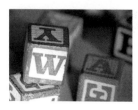

Urinary Tract

Development

The fetus excretes urine from the 12th week of intrauterine life, and by term swallows and excretes 500 mL/day. This is more important for the production of amniotic fluid than for elimination of waste products, since the fetus is being effectively haemodialysed by the placenta.

Birth demands a rapid drop in urine output. Limited excretory function is needed because body growth is rapid and milk contains exactly the right substances required for growth with little excess. When this situation is altered, the limitations of the immature kidney are seen. If the neonate has excess intravenous fluid, she becomes oedematous. If she has diarrhoea, the kidneys fail to conserve fluid adequately. Compared with the adult a relatively small decrease in renal perfusion, e.g. from mild dehydration or cardiac failure, may result in a raised plasma urea level.

Renal growth continues throughout childhood by means of increase in nephron size and not by the production of new nephrons. A steady increase of size of renal outline, as assessed by ultrasound or X-rays, is a useful sign of healthy growing kidneys.

Urine examination

Routine examination includes inspection, smell, chemical test and microscopy. Careful collection of a fresh specimen, preferably mid-stream, into a clean container is necessary. Suprapubic aspiration is easy to perform in young children (Fig. 19.1).

Inspection

Translucency
Fresh urine should appear clear when held up to the light. Chemical deposits are the commonest reason for a cloudy appearance (particularly in cold, stale urine): phosphates disappear if 2 drops of dilute acetic acid are added; urates and other acid salts dissolve on gentle warming. Infected urine is usually hazy, and can be frankly cloudy.

> If the urine appears crystal clear, it is unlikely to be infected.

Colour
The main influence on colour is the concentration, dilute urine from someone who has drunk a lot being almost colourless. Blood

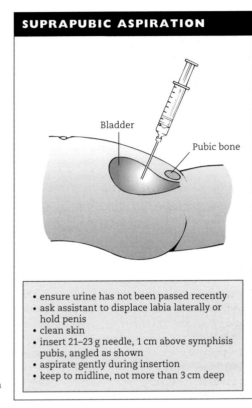

SUPRAPUBIC ASPIRATION

Bladder

Pubic bone

- ensure urine has not been passed recently
- ask assistant to displace labia laterally or hold penis
- clean skin
- insert 21–23 g needle, 1 cm above symphisis pubis, angled as shown
- aspirate gently during insertion
- keep to midline, not more than 3 cm deep

Fig. 19.1 Suprapubic aspiration of urine.

may appear obviously red but more commonly appears pinkish or reddish-brown sometimes with a 'smoky' tint. Ingested foods (e.g. beetroot), confectionery and drugs (e.g. rifampicin) are common reasons for unusual colours.

Frothiness

When the container is shaken gently, normal urine settles fast without much froth. Frothiness is a feature of protein or bile in the urine.

Smell

In some urine infections, urea-splitting organisms produce a foul fishy smell. This is also the smell of stale urine that has been left standing in a warm place. Some foods

and drugs produce characteristic odours (e.g. penicillin). Chemicals produced by body metabolism also influence urine smell: ketones commonly. Rare inborn errors of metabolism may produce characteristic odours (p. 215).

Chemical tests

The most convenient are the chemically impregnated test strips (dipstix) (OSCE, p. 200). These should be used according to the directions on the packet. The strip is immersed momentarily in the urine, the surplus urine is dislodged by tapping it and the colour change of the indicator paper is noted at the stipulated time. That time interval is critical for some tests, e.g. haemoglobin. It is important to check that the strip is held the right way round to compare appropriately with the label on the container.

Albumin

A trace of albumin is normal: 5% of children have 1+ (0.3 g/L) or more. Often this is the result of a particularly concentrated sample of urine being tested. If succeeding samples have 1+ or more albuminuria a quantitative estimation must be made by estimating the protein : creatinine ratio. Transient albuminuria may occur with fever or hard exercise. Persistent albuminuria is a feature of nephritis and kidney damage.

Glucose

Likely causes are a low renal threshold or hyperglycaemia (e.g. diabetes mellitus). In the first 2 weeks of life, small amounts of glucose and other reducing sugars are commonly found in the urine.

Haemoglobin

Even though the test is extremely sensitive and may be positive when there is no tint of blood on inspection positive reactions are abnormal. The usual cause is haematuria. Since haemoglobinuria and myoglobinuria produce a positive test also, microscopy is mandatory to identify red cells.

pH

The usual pH is 5 or 6. Alkaline urine is more likely in infants than in older children because of the frequent feeds: it also occurs after alkaline medicines and sometimes in the presence of urine infection.

Ketones

Ketonuria is common in children who are ill, anorexic or have been vomiting, or in the many schoolchildren who have had no breakfast.

Nitrite

Many urine infections are associated with excess nitrite.

Leucocytes

Excess (+ or more) may be the result of any inflammation, including infection.

Microscopy

Regardless of the precise method used, microscopic examination of urine is a most valuable skill. Some people use a counting chamber in order to record the number of formed elements per mm^3 of unspun urine. Others centrifuge the urine and enumerate it (less accurately) per high power field. There is no reliable standard for converting cells per high-power field of centrifuged urine to cells per mm^3 of unspun urine. The urine should be examined under low power with low illumination before increasing the illumination to examine under high power.

White blood cells (WBC, pus cells)

A healthy boy may have up to 5 WBC/mm^3 and a girl up to 50/mm^3. Excess cells (pyuria) may be the result of a urine infection or inflammation of the renal tract.

Red blood cells

Red blood cells (RBC) may be difficult to identify because they quickly lose their round shape and haemolyse. Urine should not contain more than 2 RBC/mm^3. The commonest causes of haematuria are glomerulonephritis and urinary tract infection.

Casts

These are formed in the renal tubules. Cellular casts may be composed of renal tubular cells, but more commonly are composed of red cells, or disintegrating red cells (granular casts). They are an important sign of glomerulonephritis. Hyaline casts devoid of cells are invariably present whenever there is proteinuria.

Bacteria

If the urine is infected bacteria can usually be seen as motile rods.

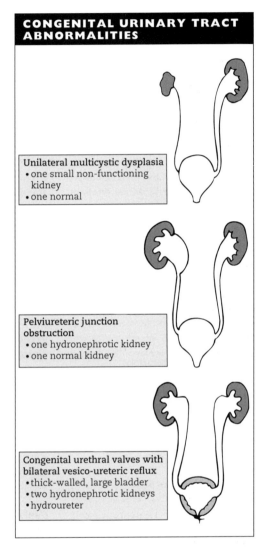

CONGENITAL URINARY TRACT ABNORMALITIES

Unilateral multicystic dysplasia
- one small non-functioning kidney
- one normal

Pelviureteric junction obstruction
- one hydronephrotic kidney
- one normal kidney

Congenital urethral valves with bilateral vesico-ureteric reflux
- thick-walled, large bladder
- two hydronephrotic kidneys
- hydroureter

Fig. 19.2 Congenital urinary tract abnormalities.

Congenital anomalies

Fetal ultrasound provides warning of many renal abnormalities. Renal agenesis, urethral valves and other obstructive lesions are detected (Fig. 19.2).

Agenesis

The ureteric bud fails to develop so that the ureter and kidney are absent. If unilateral, the child may live a healthy life provided the other kidney is normal. Bilateral agenesis is lethal; oligohydramnios is noted during pregnancy, and affected infants have pulmonary hypoplasia and characteristic facial appearance (*Potter's syndrome*).

Hypoplastic kidneys

The small kidneys are deficient in renal

parenchyma. They are not usually associated with other abnormalities.

Dysplastic kidneys

These contain abnormally differentiated parenchyma. They are commonly associated with obstruction and other abnormalities of the urinary tract. *Polycystic disease* represents one form of renal dysplasia. Infantile polycystic disease is associated with massive kidneys, renal failure early in life and a recessive pattern of inheritance, whereas adult polycystic disease which has a dominant inheritance is generally not detected in early life because the kidneys are not enlarged and function well during childhood.

Ureteric abnormalities

Obstruction is commonest at the pelvi-ureteric junction where it may cause hydronephrosis and permanent renal damage. Duplication of the ureter and pelvis may occur on one or both sides. If it only affects the upper half of the ureter, it is not important, but if it extends down to the bladder with two separate ureteric openings abnormalities of the lower ureter are common. A *ureterocele* is a cystic enlargement of the ureter within the bladder which may cause obstruction.

Bladder and urethral abnormalities

Posterior urethral valves

These are an important cause of obstruction to urine flow and occur almost exclusively in boys. They are usually detected antenatally, or present in early infancy, as acute obstruction or chronic partial obstruction with dribbling micturition.

Obstruction may cause direct damage by back pressure or predispose to urinary tract infection which may cause further damage. Most obstructive abnormalities can be corrected by surgery. Obstruction

of the lower urinary tract is frequently associated with renal dysplasia.

Hypospadias

The urethral opening is on the ventral surface of the penis. If it is at the junction of the glans and shaft, no treatment is needed, but if it is on the shaft of the penis plastic surgery is required. The foreskin may be needed for this reconstruction. In all but the mildest cases, there is ventral flexion (*chordee*) of the penis. There may be associated meatal stenosis (Fig. 19.3).

Boys with hypospadias should not be circumcised.

Renal disease

Terminology

CLASSIFICATION SYSTEM

- SYNDROMES: collection of symptoms and signs e.g. acute nephritic syndrome, nephrotic syndrome
- PATHOLOGY: results of biopsy, e.g. proliferative glomerulonephritis, minimal changes
- AETIOLOGY: e.g. diabetic, poststreptococcal

Whilst there are certain correlations between these three levels of diagnosis, it is essential to realize that a particular pathological appearance (for instance, proliferative glomerulonephritis) may be found in each of several different clinical syndromes. Further, a syndrome may be associated with several different morphological pictures, and have several different aetiologies.

The most important syndromes of renal disease in childhood are:

- acute nephritic syndrome
- recurrent haematuria

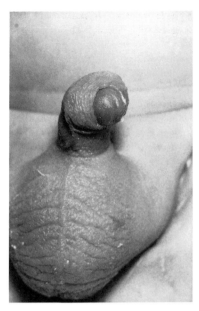

Fig. 19.3 Hypospadias. The meatus is at the junction of the glans and shaft.

- nephrotic syndrome
- symptomless proteinuria
- urinary tract infection
- renal insufficiency

Acute nephritic syndrome

- Haematuria
- Oliguria
- Hypertension
- Raised serum creatinine

Aetiology

The best-known form is *poststreptococcal glomerulonephritis*, sometimes called *acute nephritis*. The child has had a beta-haemolytic streptococcal infection, usually a pharyngitis, 2–3 weeks previously. Immune complexes composed of streptococci, antibody and complement are deposited in the glomeruli. There they provoke proliferation of the endothelial cells

(proliferative glomerulonephritis). Post-streptococcal glomerulonephritis has become rare in developed countries, but is common worldwide.

An acute nephritic syndrome may also occur at the time of pneumococcal pneumonia, septicaemia, glandular fever and other viral infections. It is sometimes seen in Henoch–Schönlein syndrome and the collagen diseases.

Features

Acute nephritic syndrome has an age distribution with a peak at 7 years. The child is well until the sudden onset of illness and the appearance of bright red or brownish urine. Facial oedema, particularly of the eyelids, is common, and there may be abdominal or loin pain together with loin tenderness. The blood pressure is usually raised.

Investigations

A small volume of blood-stained urine is passed. In addition to copious red blood cells there is an excess of white cells and proteinuria. Red cell and granular casts are present. The serum creatinine is raised in two thirds of children. If the cause is streptococcal, ASO titre is raised and serum complement is reduced.

Course and treatment

Oliguria lasts for only a few days. Diuresis usually occurs within a week and is accompanied by return of serum creatinine and blood pressure to normal. The haematuria and proteinuria gradually subside over the next year.

During the oliguric phase, fluid and protein are restricted, but it is rarely necessary to start a strict renal failure regime. Penicillin is given for 3 months to reduce the chance of recurrence, which is rare. Other treatment is symptomatic.

Over 80% make a full recovery, but a few develop progressive renal disease.

Recurrent haematuria syndrome

- Episodes of haematuria
- Association with exercise, or systemic infection
- Red cell and granular casts in the urine

The bouts of haematuria usually occur at the time of a systemic infection or exertion. The haematuria results from nephritis of unknown cause. The child may feel unwell but more often has no symptoms. The urine contains red cell and granular casts.

Between attacks the urine is normal or shows microscopic haematuria. Proteinuria is less common and may indicate more serious renal disease.

Investigations are done to exclude other causes of haematuria: urine culture, ultrasound scan and X-ray for a tumour or stone, and screening tests for bleeding disorders.

A small minority have serious and progressive nephritis, but most have a good prognosis. Their renal function is normal and continues so.

The bouts of haematuria may continue for several years, and the doctor who has the task of reassuring the parents usually ends up wishing that blood was colourless. Prolonged restriction of activity or bedrest is more likely to result in an uneducated, delinquent adolescent than to affect the renal prognosis.

Nephrotic syndrome

- Heavy proteinuria
- Hypo-albuminaemia
- Oedema

Features

Peak onset is between the ages of 2 and 5 years. Apart from the gradual onset of generalized oedema, the child may be only mildly off colour. Other symptoms are directly related to oedema, for instance discomfort from ascites or breathlessness from pleural effusion (Fig. 19.4).

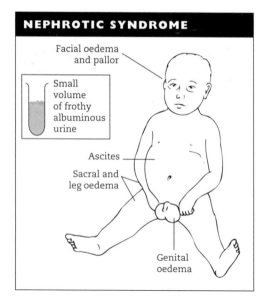

NEPHROTIC SYNDROME

Facial oedema and pallor

Small volume of frothy albuminous urine

Ascites

Sacral and leg oedema

Genital oedema

Fig. 19.4 Nephrotic syndrome.

Aetiology

Over 90% of childhood nephrotic syndrome is the result of primary renal disease of unknown cause. Nephrotic syndrome secondary to systemic illness is less common than in adults, the least rare cause being Henoch–Schönlein syndrome (p. 176). In Africa, quartan malaria is an important cause.

Pathology

Up to the age of 5 years, over 80% of affected children will show only 'minimal changes', this means that the biopsy reveals no significant abnormality. After the age of 10, more serious pathology becomes likely.

Investigations

The urine is frothy and there is heavy albuminuria. Highly selective proteinuria, that is urine containing a high proportion of small molecular weight proteins, is a good prognostic feature suggesting minimal change histology. Hyaline casts are abundant. Serum albumin is below 25 g/L and the serum cholesterol is usually raised. Serum creatinine is usually normal (Table 19.1).

Treatment and prognosis

Corticosteroids are given in large doses for 4 weeks. While there is oedema, fluid and salt are restricted: diuretics may be needed if the oedema is causing symptoms. Most children go into remission within 2 weeks of starting steroids. Diuresis occurs and the oedema and albuminuria disappear rapidly. A large proportion relapse within the next year. They can be given further courses of steroids, but if the relapses are frequent cyclophosphamide will usually produce a longer remission.

The long-term prognosis is good. Although frequent relapses can be most troublesome during childhood, with increasing age they become less frequent and most children grow out of the condition by the time they are adults and thereafter retain normal renal function and good health. A few (mainly those initially unresponsive to steroids) develop renal insufficiency.

Symptomless proteinuria

Persistent proteinuria of more than 0.3 g/day.

Table 19.1 Comparison of acute nephritic syndrome and nephrotic syndrome.

ACUTE NEPHRITIC AND NEPHROTIC SYNDROMES

	Acute nephritic syndrome	Nephrotic syndrome
Child		
Oedema	Mild facial	Gross
Blood pressure	Raised	Normal
Urine		
Albumin	++	++++
RBC	++++	0 or +
WBC	++	0
Casts	Cellular/granular	Hyaline
Bacteria	0	0
Serum		
Albumin	Normal	Low

Proteinuria is a sign of renal disease and requires investigation. Before embarking on elaborate tests of renal function or a biopsy, it is important to exclude *postural proteinuria* (orthostatic), since this is commonest between 10 and 15 years. Such children do not have proteinuria when recumbent in bed, but have excess proteinuria when up and active, particularly after adopting an excessively lordotic position. Postural proteinuria is generally considered a benign condition which does not progress.

Urinary tract infection

Incidence
From birth to adolescence the prevalence of urinary tract infection (UTI) is just over 1%. In the neonatal period, boys are more often infected, but thereafter girls predominate (25 times more likely). By the age of 2 years, 5% of girls have had a urinary tract infection.

Pathology
The commonest pathogen is *Escherichia coli*. Bacteria of the same strain are usually present in the child's gut and it is assumed that the organism enters the urethra via the perineum.

Features
In the neonate the symptoms may be non-specific — vomiting, fever or prolonged jaundice. Most children will have an infection confined to the lower urinary tract *(cystitis)* which causes merely dysuria, urgency or wetting without significant systemic illness. However, with upper tract involvement *(pyelonephritis)* illness with fever and loin pain is common.

Investigations
On inspection, the urine has an opalescent cloudy sheen. Dipstix tests are usually positive for nitrite and leucocytes and there may be haematuria and albuminuria. Motile bacteria are visible on microscopy in addition to excess white cells.

If the urine looks crystal clear and is negative for blood, nitrite and leucocytes, infection is most unlikely. If one or more of these tests is positive, the sample should be cultured. The cleanest, freshest urine sample possible should be collected, which may be difficult in infants. Self-adhesive perineal plastic bags are widely used. Suprapubic aspiration may be needed (p. 189).

Management

Initial treatment
Fluid intake is increased and frequent micturition encouraged. Appropriate chemotherapy is given: trimethoprim or nitrofurantoin are used widely. There is increasing evidence that a 1-day course (or even just one large dose) is as effective as a longer course for uncomplicated infections. For complicated or presumed *upper* tract infection prompt treatment with broad-spectrum systemic antibiotic is needed.

INTERPRETING CULTURES	
Culture result	Interpretation
<10 000 organisms/mL	Normal
10 000–100 000 organisms/mL	Unsure, therefore repeat
>100 000 organisms/mL	Urinary tract infection
Mixed growth	Contamination

Table 19.2 Interpreting urine cultures.

Further investigation

A renal ultrasound scan and abdominal X-ray should be done on any child who has had a definite urinary infection. The aim is to detect obstructive abnormalities. This is followed by further radiology if necessary. A voiding cystourethrogram is an unpleasant investigation which will define urethral abnormalities and vesico-ureteric reflux. DMSA scan identifies renal scars and provides differential renal function. Vesicoureteric reflux is present in a quarter of children with urine infection, but minor degrees of reflux in which a wisp of urine is seen to pass through the lower part of the ureter are unimportant. When there is major reflux, the urine refluxes up the ureter filling and distending the calyces, and at the end of micturition falls back to form a stagnant pool. Reflux is commoner in children than in adults, and, providing recurrent infections can be prevented, for instance by prophylactic antibiotics, it tends to go as the child grows. If medical treatment is unsuccessful, surgical correction of the reflux is possible.

Follow-up is an important part of the management. One-third of children will have a recurrence within the next year. The child's urine must be cultured a few days after completing the initial therapy and at least once in the next 3 months, *even though the child is symptomless.*

The problem of prognosis

Infection of the renal parenchyma may cause permanent or progressive damage leading to renal insufficiency. But most children with urinary tract infection do not incur renal damage. Renal damage is most likely in those with associated obstruction of the urinary tract, and in those who have severe infection and gross reflux early in life—under the age of 2. For the vast number of girls who have recurrent infections with or without symptoms during their

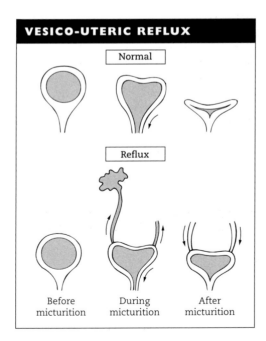

Fig. 19.5 Vesico-ureteric reflux (shown by micturating cystogram). At the end of micturition a puddle of stagnant urine remains in the bladder.

VESICO-UTERIC REFLUX

Normal

Reflux

| Before micturition | During micturition | After micturition |

school days serious renal damage is unlikely. It is sufficiently rare for some experts to suggest that treatment of *symptomless* urine infection is not necessary.

Renal calculi

Stones in the urinary tract of children are less common than in adults. Occasionally they cause pain or renal colic but more often are detected by chance on X-ray. Most stones are of infective origin, especially in boys with a proteus infection. Since they can be of metabolic origin it is customary to check the urine for abnormal amino acids (e.g. cystinuria) and the serum calcium and phosphate.

Renal insufficiency (renal failure)

Acute renal failure

Acute renal failure describes the situation in which previously healthy kidneys suddenly stop working. It is a rewarding condition to treat in childhood because a high proportion of children have recoverable conditions that present acutely such as acute tubular necrosis in hypovolaemic shock.

A particularly notorious form is the *haemolytic–uraemic syndrome* (HUS) which affects mainly older infants and toddlers who have been infected with verotoxin producing *E. coli* O157. After a brief gastroenteritis-like illness the child presents with a haemolytic anaemia, thrombocytopenia and acute renal failure. Early peritoneal dialysis and expert management in a paediatric renal unit enable more than 80% to recover completely.

Chronic renal failure

Progressive renal insufficiency or *chronic renal failure* is uncommon. During the early months of life, congenital abnormalities,

particularly renal dysplasia, are the main cause. Thereafter various forms of glomerulonephritis are the commonest cause. Children with end stage renal disease have the same features as adults, e.g. anaemia, hypertension and renal rickets: in addition they fail to grow.

Successful transplantation is the aim, and results for children are better than for adults. Until transplantation is possible the child is maintained on dialysis: continuous/intermittent ambulatory peritoneal dialysis is frequently used despite the common complication of peritonitis.

Male genitalia

Undescended testicles

The testicles normally descend into the scrotum about the 36th week of gestation and are therefore usually fully descended in the newborn full-term infant. Spontaneous descent may occur later, but the older the child the less likely is this to happen. If a testis remains undescended until after puberty, it will not mature properly and will be sterile. 'Undescended' testicles are often incompletely descended and are palpable in the inguinal canal. If such a testis cannot be persuaded into the scrotum, or if the testis cannot be felt at all, orchidopexy is advised.

Incompletely descended testes need to be distinguished from retractile testes and ectopic testes. Retractile testes are very common and normal. An active cremaster muscle will withdraw the testis into the inguinal canal or higher, especially if the doctor has cold hands. Ectopic testes are rare and may be located in the superficial inguinal pouch, near the femoral ring, or in the perineum.

Hydrocele

At birth it is quite common to find fluid in the scrotal sac. It almost always clears up without treatment. In older infants and children there may be a tense hydrocele on one or both sides. It does not cause symptoms but is often associated with inguinal hernia. Surgery is therefore advised.

Circumcision

The foreskin is normally adherent to the glans in the early months of life and sometimes for as long as 3 or 4 years. In infancy therefore the foreskin can only be retracted by breaking down the adhesions, a procedure that is unnecessary for the baby and distressing for the parents. A non-retractile prepuce in early life is not an indication for circumcision. If the preputial orifice is small enough to obstruct urine flow *(phimosis)*, circumcision is indicated. In *paraphimosis*, the tight foreskin is retracted behind the glans penis and cannot be returned. If reduction is not possible with anaesthesia, an emergency dorsal slit followed later by circumcision may be needed.

Posthitis (inflammation of the foreskin) is common in babies while they are still in nappies. It requires treating as for nappy rash and is a contraindication to circumcision because of the risk of a meatal ulcer. If normal separation of the foreskin from the glans does not occur by about the third year of life, or if the foreskin cannot be retracted in order to clean underneath, then *balanitis* (inflammation of the glans) may occur and may be an indication for circumcision.

Jews and Muslims require their boys to be circumcised.

Female genitalia

Adherent labia minora

Sometimes firm adhesions develop between opposing surfaces of the labia minora, probably as a consequence of poor personal hygiene. Urine is passed normally, but the appearance may suggest that there is no vaginal orifice. The labia may be separated with a probe or repeated application of oestrogen cream.

When having their perineum examined, young girls are likely to be happiest if lying supine on their mother's lap or on a couch with their legs up in the lithotomy position. They can see what the examiner is up to. The labia are gently pulled apart to check that they are not adherent and the vulva is inspected. Vaginal examination should be performed by those with expertise.

Vaginal discharge

Soreness and irritation of the vulva in girls is usually due to lack of personal hygiene. Micturition may be painful. Staining of the pants may result from normal heavy secretion of mucus particularly about puberty. Careful daily washing and drying of the perineum will relieve both conditions. A purulent vaginal discharge is less common.

Pus should be cultured and examined for *Trichomonas* and other sexually transmitted disease. The possibility of sexual abuse or an underlying foreign body should be borne in mind.

CAUSES OF VAGINAL DISCHARGE

- White mucoid (leucorrhoea)
  - In neonate, normal
  - At puberty, normal

- Offensive yellow (vulvovaginitis)
  - Aged 2–5 years, associated with poor hygiene
  - Infection
  - Sexual abuse
  - Foreign body

- Bloody (vaginal bleeding)
  - In neonate may be normal
  - Sexual abuse
  - Foreign body
  - Tumour

- Menarche

OSCE Station: Urine testing

Clinical approach:

Check
- name and date on sample
- any clinical information given

Inspection
- appearance
  ◊ clear/cloudy/hazy
  ◊ red: blood, dietary pigment, drugs
  ◊ frothy: high protein content
- smell
  ◊ musty: infection, old specimen
  ◊ abnormal smell: dietary; inborn error of metabolism

Reagent strip urinalysis
- pH: usual range pH 5–7
- blood: normally negative; trace may be normal
- protein: normal = negative or trace; scored: + to ++++
- specific gravity: varies with hydration, and renal function; usually 1.010–1.020
- glucose: normally negative; scored: trace to ++++
- ketones: found in starvation, diabetes etc.
- nitrite: larger amounts associated with infection
- leucocytes: larger amounts associated with infection

A 3-year-old girl presents with fever and vomiting. Please test her urine

- shake gently, and hold up to light

The urine appears slightly hazy, and has a musty unpleasant smell

- immerse a reagent stick in the urine and remove
- tap excess urine from the stick
- hold stick horizontally and start timing
- read colour reaction at times indicated on label of bottle

This urine shows:
pH 8
blood: trace
protein: +
nitrite: positive
leucocytes: large

> The findings are typical of a urine infection.

Never forget:

- find the container that the dipstix came in and read instructions on it
- the reagent stick must be lined up with the key printed on the container for interpretation
- make sure the stick is the right way up!
- reagents react at different times: it is important to time this test

Look around for:

- clinical notes, growth charts

Special points

- interpret your observations in the light of any clinical history
- always consider urine infection in acutely ill children
- consider whether any laboratory investigation is needed (e.g. urine culture)
- urinalysis 'dipstix' vary in the number of reagents on each stick
- do not do this for the first time in the undergraduate examination

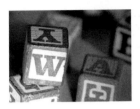

Haematology

The normal blood picture

The full-term infant has a haemoglobin of 17 g/dL (range 14–20). Limited erythropoiesis and red cell survival leads to a fall in the haemoglobin level until 3 months. Red cell size (MCV) is large at birth, low at 1 year and rises to the adult level at puberty. Low MCV is seen in iron deficiency and thalassaemia trait.

At birth haemoglobin is mainly of the fetal type — HbF (Fig. 20.1). HbF is gradually replaced by HbA. Children have high white cell count and lymphocytes count, particularly in the first year. Infection often provokes a marked neutrophil leukocytosis with immature white cells pouring out of the marrow (a shift to the left). In infants, a lymphocytic response to infection does not exclude a bacterial cause.

The platelet count is slightly reduced in the first few months but by 6 months the normal adult value of $250–350 \times 10^9$/L is reached. The ESR should be below 16, provided that the packed cell volume is at least 35%. Plasma viscosity (normal 1.5–1.7) is a satisfactory alternative to ESR.

Anaemia

Anaemia is common in childhood, but not quite as common as many mothers suspect.

Mothers worry about pallor. Children of fair complexion may be pale but not anaemic. Anaemia may cause tiredness and even breathlessness, but most tired children are not anaemic.

Anaemia may be caused by:
- diminished production of red cells
- excessive breakdown of red cells
- blood loss.

Diminished production

Deficiency anaemias

Iron deficiency anaemia is by far the most common, and is characterized by a hypochromic microcytic blood picture. Reduction in MCV is a useful early sign, and is followed by a reduction of mean corpuscular haemoglobin concentration. Basically it is caused by insufficient intake of iron, which is more common in:
- Preterm babies and twins (p. 67).
- Infants who have to exist entirely on cow's milk and are late changing to iron-containing weaning foods — sometimes because the infant is late learning to chew solids.
- Homes where poverty, ignorance, or religious/racial factors prevent the child from receiving red meat, green vegetables, eggs, and bread (which are the main sources of iron). Older infants and toddlers are most at risk.
- Chronic malabsorption.

- Adolescent girls with rapid growth and menstrual losses.

Other deficiency anaemias are uncommon. Folic acid deficiency is rare and even in coeliac disease, iron deficiency is more common. Pernicious anaemia is extremely rare in children.

Bone marrow disturbance

Infiltration. Leukaemia (p. 208) is the most important. Secondary deposits from malignant tumours is less common.

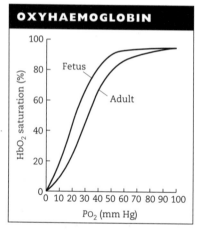

Fig. 20.1 Fetal and adult oxyhaemoglobin dissociation curves.

Toxic damage

Chronic infection or inflammation and renal insufficiency depress haemopoiesis. Aplastic anaemia may be drug related, post viral (e.g. Epstein–Barr) or more commonly idiopathic.

Excessive breakdown

Haemolytic anaemias are not common except in the newborn (p. 70). Some are specific to children and others cause their main problems in childhood. They are characterized by chronic or recurrent anaemia with slight jaundice at times. While haemolysis is active, there is usually a reticulocytosis. When the haemolysis is severe and sudden, it is called a 'haemolytic crisis'; jaundice, dark urine and dark stools are likely. Splenomegaly is a feature of chronic cases.

Cellular abnormalities

These comprise abnormalities of red cell shape, intracellular enzymes, or haemoglobin structure.

Red cell shape. The most important is *hereditary spherocytosis*. Red cells are small, spherical and show increased osmotic fragility. It is autosomal dominant, but one-third are new mutations.

Enzyme defect. The commonest is *glucose-6-phosphate dehydrogenase* (G6PD) *deficiency.*

	Haemoglobin		WBC	Lymphocytes	
Age	(g/dL)	Type	MCV	(×10⁹/L)	(%)
birth	17	HbF > HbA	96	16.00	32
1 month	15	HbF > HbA	91	11.0	50
3 months	11	HbF < HbA	84	11.0	50
1 year	12	HbA	78	10.0	55
4 years	13	HbA	80	9.0	40
12 years	14	HbA	81	8.0	30

NORMAL BLOOD

Table 20.1 Normal blood picture.

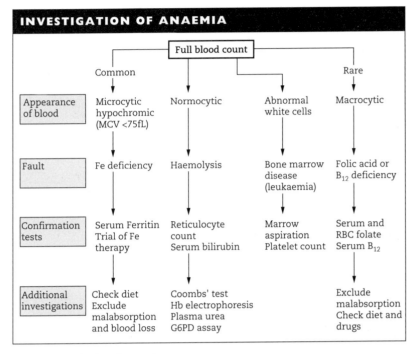

INVESTIGATION OF ANAEMIA

	Full blood count			
	Common			**Rare**
Appearance of blood	Microcytic hypochromic (MCV <75fL)	Normocytic	Abnormal white cells	Macrocytic
Fault	Fe deficiency	Haemolysis	Bone marrow disease (leukaemia)	Folic acid or B$_{12}$ deficiency
Confirmation tests	Serum Ferritin Trial of Fe therapy	Reticulocyte count Serum bilirubin	Marrow aspiration Platelet count	Serum and RBC folate Serum B$_{12}$
Additional investigations	Check diet Exclude malabsorption and blood loss	Coombs' test Hb electrophoresis Plasma urea G6PD assay		Exclude malabsorption Check diet and drugs

Fig. 20.2 Investigation of anaemia.

It is rare in Britain except in families of Mediterranean, African or Chinese origin. It is X-linked recessive.

G6PD CHILDREN SHOULD AVOID:

- Sulphonamides (e.g. cotrimoxazole)
- Quinolones (e.g. ciprofloxacin)
- Quinines (e.g. primaquine, chloroquine)
- Some broad beans (*favism*)

Haemoglobinopathies. The synthesis of haemoglobin is under genetic control. Some abnormal genes interfere with the production of entire globin chains (e.g. β chains) so that the affected person lacks normal haemoglobin (e.g. β thalassaemia). Other abnormal genes result in the substi-

tution of an amino acid in the globin chain, so producing an abnormal haemoglobin (e.g. HbS). Haemoglobin electrophoresis identifies abnormal haemoglobins and quantifies HbA and HbF.

Thalassaemia

HbA is deficient and there is persistent preponderance of HbF.

Thalassaemia occurs in a broad belt extending from the Mediterranean countries through India to the Far East (Fig. 20.3). The Mediterranean form is usually β thalassaemia. It is inherited as an autosomal recessive trait. Those with the heterozygous state have thalassaemia trait and are asymptomatic or have a mild anaemia (*thalassaemia minor*). Their red cells contain up to 20% HbF. Those with the homozygous state (*thalassaemia major*) have profound anaemia, the Hb level depending upon the

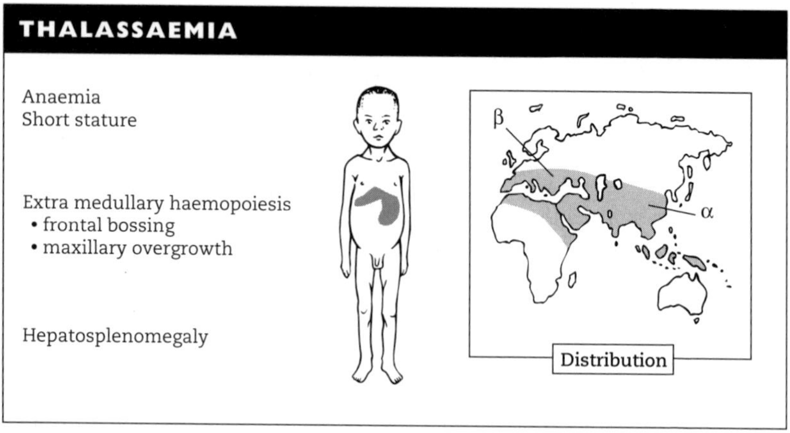

THALASSAEMIA

Anaemia
Short stature

Extra medullary haemopoiesis
• frontal bossing
• maxillary overgrowth

Hepatosplenomegaly

β

α

Distribution

Fig. 20.3 Thalassaemia major.

balance of red cell production and destruction. Sometimes an acceptable level is sustained *(thalassaemia intermedia)*. α Thalassaemia, which causes hydrops and perinatal death, occurs mainly in the Far East.

Treatment involves regular blood transfusion every 3–4 weeks to maintain the Hb level, desferrioxamine by nightly subcutaneous infusion to prevent iron overload, and supplements of folic acid and vitamin C to support red cell production. Hypersplenism may develop. Prenatal diagnosis and carrier detection are well established.

Sickle cell disease

SICKLE CELL DISEASE

• Anaemia

• Acute crises
   ♦ Painful, vaso-occlusive
   ♦ Haemolytic
   ♦ Sequestration
   ♦ Aplastic (post parvovirus)

• Infection (e.g. pneumoccus)

• Dactylitis (hand–foot syndrome)

This disorder occurs in the black races. HbS is present in place of HbA. At low oxygen tensions the cell becomes crescent or sickle-shaped and is likely to haemolyse. Heterozygotes have about 30% HbS, may show sickling, but are usually symptomless. Homozygotes develop recurrent episodes of haemolysis from infancy. Intravascular thromboses in mesenteric, intracranial or bone vessels produce severe pain, simulating acute abdominal emergencies, meningitis or arthritis. Treatment is symptomatic.

Painful crises need:
• Analgesia
• Oxygen
• Hydration
• Warmth

Prognosis is poor; many die in late childhood or early adult life from infections, cardiac failure, or thrombotic episodes. Outlook is better if general health and nutrition is good. DNA probes are available for prenatal diagnosis and carrier detection.

ⓘ Up to 25% of children with sickle cell disease die of pneumococcal infection. All should be given penicillin prophylaxis and pneumococcal vaccination.

Extracellular abnormalities

Antibodies causing premature destruction of the red cell are usually associated with a positive Coombs' test. The only common example in childhood is haemolytic disease of the newborn (p. 71). Rarer causes include severe poisoning or infection, malignancy, and systemic lupus erythematosus.

Blood loss

Hidden blood loss is not common in childhood: peptic ulcers, piles and gastrointestinal malignancy are rare. Gastrointestinal bleeding from a Meckel's diverticulum or reflux oesophagitis is more likely to present with overt bleeding than unexplained anaemia.

Coagulation disorders

Haemophilia

Presentation

• Excessive bruising as the boy learns to crawl and walk during the second year
• Prolonged bleeding following circumcision, blood sampling or tooth eruption
Haemophila A is over 5 times more common than B (Table 20.2). Severity is related to the degree of deficiency of the relevant factor. In Haemophilia A, symptoms occur with less than 10% of normal clotting activity. Severe disease occurs with <1%. Prolonged clotting time and partial thromboplastin time lead to specific assay of the relevant coagulation factor. (Prothrombin time is normal.)

Treatment

Bleeding episodes are treated by IV injection of factor concentrate; most families manage their own injections. The aim is to protect the child from trauma by forbidding contact sports, and yet encouraging an active, enjoyable life. Haemarthroses, especially of the ankle and knees, are a potential problem since recurrence can lead to permanent joint damage.

Prophylactic dental care is important. Haemorrhage after dental extraction and other surgical procedures can be avoided by admitting the child to hospital for factor replacement.

Haemophilia usually becomes less severe as an adult. Regional haemophilia centres provide expert care and provide a service for prenatal diagnosis and the identification of female carriers.

Von Willebrand's syndrome affects both boys and girls, with autosomal dominant inheritance. Though there is a combination of Factor VIII deficiency and platelet dysfunction, the degree of the bleeding disorder is usually mild.

Table 20.2 Haemophilia.

HAEMOPHILIA

Haemophilia	Deficient factor	Inheritance
A	VIII	X-linked recessive
B (Christmas disease)	IX	X-linked recessive

CAUSES OF PURPURA

Platelet count low (thrombocytopenia)	Platelet count normal
Idiopathic thrombocytopenic purpura	Septicaemia (particularly meningococcal)
Leukaemia (p. 208)	Henoch–Schönlein syndrome (p. 176)
Disseminated intravascular coagulation	Common infectious illnesses and viraemia
Toxic effect of drugs	

Table 20.3 Main causes of purpura in children.

> **i** Before 1985, some factor VIII was contaminated with HIV. Many haemophiliacs died of AIDS. All factor VIII is now treated to prevent transmission.

Thrombocytopenia

Thrombocytopenia may be a feature of several systemic diseases as well as infiltrative diseases of the bone marrow and marrow aplasia. The most common thrombocytopenic purpura of childhood is *idiopathic thrombocytopenic purpura* (ITP). The onset is acute, often occurring 1–3 weeks after an upper respiratory tract infection. A widespread petechial rash appears, developing into small purpuric spots. There may be bleeding from the nose or into the mucous membranes. Serious internal or intracranial bleeds are rare.

ITP

- Hb normal

- WBC normal

- Platelets low ($< 30 \times 10^9$/L)

- Marrow
  - ↑ Immature megakaryocytes

Generally the outcome is good. Seventy-five per cent of children make a complete recovery within a month. Transfusions of platelets and blood are rarely needed. Corticosteroids reduce the risk of massive haemorrhage. Splenectomy is reserved for the small minority who have persistent or recurrent thrombocytopenia.

> Purpuric spots do not fade when pressed.

Disseminated intravascular coagulation (DIC, consumption coagulopathy)

This syndrome is an important cause of bleeding and purpura (Table 20.3). Examination of the blood shows haemolytic anaemia, fragmented red cells, thrombocytopenia and deficiency of coagulation factors. In the neonate, it occurs as a result of severe hypoxia or massive infection. In older children, it may be associated with septicaemia and other severe illnesses.

OSCE Station: Assessment of bruising

Clinical approach:

Check
- colour
- anaemia
- jaundice

Bruising
- site
  - where are the bruises?
  - are they over bony prominences?
- character
  - small petechiae
  - large bruised areas
  - does pattern suggest mode of injury?
- age
  - bruises change appearance as they age
  - are these bruises of different ages?

Associated disease
- coagulation disorders
  - previous bleeding into joints
  - medicalert bracelet
- other haematological disorders
  - red cell problem—anaemia
  - white cell problem—ill health, infection, treatment of malignancy
- if time allows or you are asked, examine for hepatosplenomegaly, and lymphadenopathy

Sam is 5 years old. He has some marks on his skin. Please examine them

- looks well and cheerful

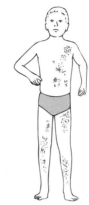

- normal growth
- widespread rash
- non-blanching
- varying size
  - petechiae and bruises
- no enlarged liver or spleen
- normal cervical nodes

Sam has idiopathic thrombocytopenic purpura (ITP).

Never forget:

- say hello and introduce yourself
- general health—is the child ill?
- colour—?pale/ ?jaundice
- quickly assess growth, nutrition, and development
- mention the obvious (e.g. drip, hair loss from chemotherapy)

Look around for:

- other injuries
- features of neglect or abuse
- treatment of associated disease
  - intravenous line
  - indwelling cannula

Special points

- non-accidental injury (NAI) is suggested by the pattern, site and varied ages of bruises
- NAI is unusual in undergraduate examinations, but you might be asked why this child's bruises do not suggest NAI
- accidental bruises are very common in childhood (usually on legs and forehead)
- accidental bruising is rare before the infant walks

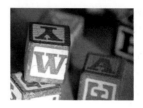

Neoplastic Disease

Malignant disease is the second commonest cause of death in childhood after accidents (Fig. 21.1). With 1200 newly diagnosed UK cases a year, a child has a 1 in 600 chance of developing a malignancy before reaching adulthood. The commonest malignancies are leukaemia, lymphoma and central nervous system tumours. In contrast to adult disease, childhood epithelial malignancies (e.g. carcinoma of the lung and gastrointestinal tract) are very rare. Furthermore, childhood tumours show a better response to therapy than adult tumours (Table 21.1).

Acute leukaemia

Leukaemia is characterized by the malignant proliferation of abnormal white cells (blasts) within the bone marrow. Acute lymphoblastic accounts for 85% of cases. It is commoner in boys and has a peak incidence between 2 and 5 years of age.

The diagnosis is confirmed by bone marrow examination. Blasts may also be seen within the peripheral blood. Children with a total white blood cell count less than 50×10^9/L at diagnosis have a good prognosis, whilst those with a count greater than 100×10^9/L have a worse outlook. Ini-

---

LEUKAEMIA PRESENTATION

- Thrombocytopenia → bruising
- Anaemia → pallor
- Leucopenia → infection

Also:
- ◆ Bone pain
- ◆ Fever
- ◆ Lymphadenopathy
- ◆ Hepatosplenomegaly

---

tial treatment consists of induction chemotherapy with the aim of achieving remission (defined as less than 5% blasts on bone marrow examination). Within 1 month of commencing chemotherapy 95% of children will achieve remission. Because meningeal leukaemia is a common complication, induction must be followed by intrathecal methotrexate, sometimes with cranial irradiation. Remission is maintained with intermittent cycles of chemotherapy for 2 years. With modern aggressive therapy, 70% of children will remain disease free 5 years after diagnosis. Relapse is rare after that time.

Children with acute myeloid leukaemia have a less favourable outcome. Remission can be achieved in 80% using intensive

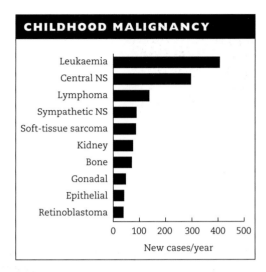

Fig. 21.1 Incidence of childhood malignancy in the UK.

SURVIVAL RATES

Malignancy	Long-term survival rate (%)
Hodgkin's lymphoma	90
Wilm's tumour	80
Astrocytoma	70
Acute lymphoblastic leukaemia	70
Osteosarcoma	50
Neuroblastoma	40
All childhood malignancy	60

Table 21.1 Long-term survival rates (%) for childhood malignancy.

chemotherapy regimens, but relapse is common. For those in remission bone marrow transplantation may offer the best chance of cure.

Lymphomas

Lymphomas are classified into two groups based on their histological characteristics.

Hodgkin's disease and Non-Hodgkin's disease has a peak incidence in young adults. Treatment is with radiotherapy and/or chemotherapy depending on the extent of the disease. The five-year survival rate is good (93%). Non-Hodgkin's lymphoma has a peak incidence between the ages of 7 and 10 years. It is almost always a generalized disease requiring treatment with intensive multiple drug chemotherapy; 70% of children will achieve prolonged remission.

Central nervous system tumours

These are most commonly gliomas: either astrocytomas or medulloblastomas. They are mainly infratentorial and present with cerebellar signs. Papilloedema is an important sign. Computer-assisted tomography or magnetic resonance imaging will identify the site and extent of the tumour.

Treatment includes surgical excision, radiotherapy and chemotherapy. Astrocytomas have the best survival rates.

Neuroblastoma

This is a malignant tumour arising from the sympathetic nervous tissue. It commonly develops within the adrenal gland, but can arise from the cervical, thoracic or lumbar sympathetic chains. The commonest presentation is with an abdominal mass. Early metastasis to bone, liver and skin often occurs. Urinary levels of catecholamine degradation products (e.g. VMA, HMMA) are usually raised.

Treatment comprises chemotherapy combined with radiotherapy and surgery. The outlook is poor except for those presenting with localized disease and for children aged less than 1 year.

Wilms' tumour (nephroblastoma)

Nephroblastomas are embryonic renal tumours which usually present as a unilateral abdominal mass during early childhood. The mass is often solid and cystic within the kidney. Microscopic haematuria occurs in up to one-third of cases, but macroscopic haematuria is rare. Surgical excision and chemotherapy often achieve complete cure.

Bone tumours

Ewing's sarcoma and osteosarcoma usually occur in the long bones and present with pain, swelling or a pathological fracture. Treatment is aimed at surgical excision of the tumour, followed by endoprosthetic replacement of the bone and joint, thereby avoiding amputation. Chemotherapy is given before and after surgery. Radiotherapy may also be required. Half the children achieve long-term survival.

Treatment of childhood malignancy

The improvements in the treatment and survival of childhood malignancy have been dramatic over the last 30 years. As survival increases, the adverse effects of treatment become more apparent. In the short term, chemotherapy and radiotherapy may lead to bone marrow suppression resulting in an increased risk of infection and the requirement for supportive care with blood products.

A small proportion of survivors later develop a second primary tumour. Social and psychological problems for the child, their siblings and the family are inevitable. The diversity and complications of treatment mandates treatment in a specialized centre where there is a multidisciplinary team. Long-term follow-up is important. For the child whose disease cannot be cured, every effort should be made for palliative care to be given at home or within a children's hospice.

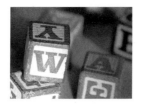

Endocrine and Metabolic Disorders

Insulin-dependent diabetes mellitus is the most important endocrine condition in children. Other hormonal conditions, and inborn errors of metabolism, are relatively uncommon, and most are extremely rare. In general they are characterized by their effects upon a child's growth and development. It is important therefore to include endocrine and metabolic disorders in the differential diagnosis of a wide variety of clinical presentations. Early recognition and appropriate management may confer long-lasting benefit.

Diabetes mellitus

Diabetes in children is almost exclusively insulin dependent. It has increased in frequency, now affecting around 1:500 children. Most present after the age of 2 years. Other members of the family may have diabetes or other autoimmune disease. Children who are genetically predisposed develop diabetes following an unknown environmental trigger. Possible triggers include viral infection and cow's milk protein.

Presentation

> ### PRESENTING FEATURES OF DIABETES MELLITUS
>
> - Polydipsia/thirst
> - Polyuria/enuresis
> - Weight loss
> - Dehydration/vomiting
> - Ketoacidosis
> - Altered consciousness/coma

At presentation, children are often ill and have a markedly elevated blood glucose level (>14 mmol/L), together with glycosuria and ketonuria. The glucose tolerance test is hardly ever used in children. The HbA_{1C} may be useful for diagnosis and for monitoring.

Management

The principles of management of ketoacidosis are rehydration, control of blood sugar and care of electrolyte status. Management involves principally the introduction of dietary and insulin therapy, and an intensive programme of support and education for the child and their family.

> If diabetes mellitus is suspected, or glycosuria is found, check blood sugar with a stick test: if the blood sugar is elevated, refer immediately.

MANAGEMENT OF DIABETES MELLITUS

Aims
- Regulated carbohydrate intake matching growth needs and activity
- Insulin regime designed around child and family's needs and abilities
- Continuous monitoring of control — usually home blood glucose

Advice to family
- Understanding of blood sugar control
- Good control reduces likelihood of complications
- Diabetes management can usually be adjusted round lifestyle
- How to adjust diet/insulin with activity/illness
- Recognition, importance and treatment of hypoglycaemia

There is a wide variety of different insulin preparations. Most children begin on a twice-daily regime with a mixture of short- and medium-acting insulin. Some teenagers prefer a multidose regime using one of the pen devices, which allows greater flexibility, but demands a high level of understanding on the part of the teenager. Insulin is injected subcutaneously, rotating round sites including the arms, thighs and abdomen.

Each child will get different early symptoms of hypoglycaemia. It is essential that they understand the importance of recognizing a 'hypo'. The child may wear a medical alert bracelet. The family, teachers and others caring for the child should understand that whenever the child becomes acutely unwell, the administration of a small amount of sugary food or drink is always the right thing to do. If a child is unable to eat or drink, sugar or jam can be smeared on to the buccal mucosa and is rapidly absorbed. The child's parents should know how to administer subcutaneous or intramuscular glucagon in emergencies.

Diabetic control can be difficult in children. Loss of control during infection, and difficulty in maintaining tight control during periods of rapid growth, are characteristic.

Family support

All children with diabetes, and their families, require intensive support. Children should be encouraged, as soon as they are old enough, to take responsibility for their diabetes. Membership of Diabetes UK is a great asset. Self-help groups and the outreach children's nursing service can all help the child and the family to take diabetes in their stride, so that it is not a major interference with the normal way of life. Children with diabetes tend to be somewhat late in puberty. Long-term complications, such as retinopathy and renal disease, are rare during childhood.

Chronic illness does not fit well into the teenage years. This is well known in diabetes, when depression and psychological disturbance become more common. The discipline of diabetes is particularly irksome at this age. Teenagers should be encouraged to become more independent of their parents, managing their own diabetes. Unfortunately they may frequently break dietary rules, cheat on tests or omit insulin.

Hypoglycaemia

Hypoglycaemia is most common in the newborn period. Symptoms are difficult to recognize in babies, and routine monitoring is indicated for those at high risk (p. 71).

Hypoglycaemia should be excluded in all children who become acutely ill. If a child collapses, blood glucose is the first thing to measure.

If hypoglycaemia is allowed to persist, permanent neurological damage may occur. This may lead to cerebral palsy, learning problems and epilepsy. In the collapsed child, intravenous dextrose is given. Investigation is complex.

CAUSES OF HYPOGLYCAEMIA

- Hormonal
  - Excess insulin
  - Lack of cortisol (e.g. congenital adrenal hyperplasia)

- Metabolic
  - Ketotic hypoglycaemia
  - Liver disease
  - Glycogen storage disorders
  - Galactosaemia
  - Other inborn errors of metabolism

Thyroid disease

Normal thyroid function is necessary for healthy physical and mental growth.

Congenital hypothyroidism

This is usually due to the absence of the thyroid gland. Occasionally a small or ectopic thyroid is present, or metabolic problems in the gland prevent production of thyroid hormone. Neonatal screening at the end of the first week of life allows detection of the TSH, which is raised. Very rarely hypothyroidism is due to panhypopituitarism and TSH levels are normal.

This successful screening programme allows early instigation of lifelong hormone replacement therapy with oral thyroxine.

Without treatment, congenital hypothyroidism results in *cretinism*. The dwarfed child with coarse features, scanty hair, an umbilical hernia and severe learning problems is now a feature of history.

Juvenile hypothyroidism

Later thyroid failure is more common in children with diabetes and in those with Down's or Turner's syndromes. Features are very similar to those seen in the adult, although school failure and learning problems are more frequently recognized. The cardinal features is a fall-off in physical growth (p. 88). Juvenile hypothyroidism is normally due to auto-immune disease and auto-antibodies are present. Rarely it is of pituitary origin.

Hyperthyroidism and goitre

A transient form of this occurs in newborn infants who receive IgG transplacentally from a mother who has a history of *Graves' disease* (autoimmune hyperthyroidism often associated with exophthalmos). This condition is transient.

Goitre may occur in adolescent girls who are euthyroid. Classical Graves' disease is unusual in children.

The adrenal glands

Disorders of the adrenal gland are uncommon in children. The least rare is congenital adrenal hyperplasia (adrenogenital syndrome). *Addison's disease* (hypoadrenalism), presenting later in life with growth failure and hyperpigmentation, is very rare. Cushing's syndrome is the result of excess corticosteroids activity, and is almost always the result of therapeutic use of steroids. Rarely, adrenal cortical tumours secrete androgens or oestrogens, with consequent early appearance of secondary sexual characteristics (adrenarche).

Congenital adrenal hyperplasia

This results from a metabolic block in the synthesis of hydrocortisone. The 21-hydroxylase enzyme is absent in children who are homozygous for an autosomal recessive gene mutation. There are two consequences:

• absence of sufficient circulating corticosteroids and mineralocorticoids
• excess production of adrenal cortical hormone caused by increased production of ACTH by the pituitary.

Clinical features depend on the child's sex. Girls are virilized with abnormal genitalia, enlarged clitoris and labia fusion which may prevent accurate determination of sex at birth. Boys have normal genitalia. The majority of children with this condition lack mineralocorticoids, and present in the first weeks because of salt loss. Typically they have a history of vomiting and are markedly dehydrated. Some are severely ill and the condition is lethal if not recognized and treated.

Diagnosis is made by finding elevated levels of cortisone precursors and, in salt losers, a low serum sodium and an elevated potassium. Treatment is lifelong hormone replacement therapy. The dose must be increased at times of illness and stress. Girls may require genital, plastic surgery.

> If a newborn infant is not clearly male or female do not ascribe the sex. This is awkward, but better than discovering that a boy is in fact a girl.

Cushing's syndrome

FEATURES OF CUSHING'S SYNDROME

- Round, fat face
- Obesity
- Poor growth
- Hypertension
- Osteoporosis

The effects of excess glucocorticoid are almost always due to steroid treatment. Long-term steroid therapy should only be used when it is essential. *Cushing's disease* (primary excess steroid secretion by the child's own adrenals), and other causes of endogenous excess glucocorticoids, are

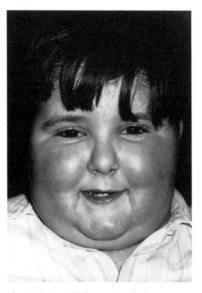

Fig. 22.1 Steroid therapy has led to obesity, a round face and hirsuteness.

rare. The combination of obesity and reduced height/growth should raise suspicion (Fig. 22.1).

Growth hormone deficiency

Defiency of growth hormone (GH) is an uncommon, but important, cause of growth failure. It may be isolated, or associated with deficiency of other pituitary hormones. It is sometimes secondary to an intracranial lesion.

Diagnosis depends upon demonstrating a lack of response to stimulation of growth hormone secretial. This test is combined with other hormone assays. GH secretion is stimulated by clonidine or glucagon and blood samples are taken over a few hours.

Genetically engineered human GH is given by injection, under expert supervision and close monitoring. GH has also been used to treat short children without deficiency (e.g. Turner's syndrome, achondroplasia). *Creutzfeldt–Jakob disease* occurs in a small number of GH treated children from the time when cadaveric GH was used from 1958 to 1985.

Diabetes insipidus

This rare disease results from either failure of the hypothalamus to produce sufficient antidiuretic hormone (ADH) or failure of the renal tubule to respond to it (nephrogenic diabetes insipidus). There is marked thirst, and the passage of large volumes of dilute urine of low osmolality. There is constant danger of serious water depletion, especially in hot weather.

ADH deficiency can result from brain tumours, cysts, vascular accidents and meningitis. ADH replacement therapy is given. Nephrogenic DI is caused by an X-linked gene and therefore only occurs in males.

Inborn errors of metabolism

There are many hundreds of these disorders due a metabolic block. Most are extremely rare, and most show autosomal recessive inheritance (Fig. 22.2).

SYMPTOMS WHICH SUGGEST AN INBORN ERROR OF METABOLISM

- Unexplained illness
- Fits, coma
- Hypoglycaemia, metabolic acidosis
- Acute liver disease; jaundice
- Failure to thrive
- Developmental delay

Diagnosis is made by collecting urine, preferably at the time of symptoms, for a 'metabolic screen'. Successful management usually depends upon dietary restriction or replacement of the missing metabolites. Many of the severe inborn errors of metabolism are not amenable to treatment.

Phenylketonuria (PKU)

This disorder affects 1 : 10 000–20 000 children born with a deficiency of the enzyme which converts phenylalanine to tyrosine. High levels of phenylalanine in the blood result in delayed development, poor growth and seizures (Table 22.1).

Children affected by PKU are detected in the neonatal screening programme (p. 61). Early implementation of a strict low pheny-

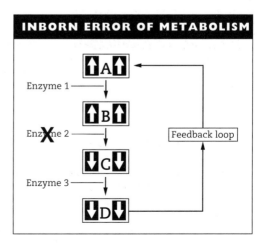

Fig. 22.2 Schematic inborn error of metabolism. Enzyme 2 is non-functional. Low levels of D provide positive feedback driving the metabolic pathway. Clinical symptoms may result from low levels of C or D OR the high levels of A or B. Diagnosis is usually made by measuring the high levels of A or B, or by determination of enzyme activity.

INBORN ERROR OF METABOLISM

Enzyme 1

Enzyme 2

Enzyme 3

Feedback loop

SCREENING CRITERIA

| Screening test criteria | Condition | |
	Hypothyroidism	Phenylketonuria
Identifiable disease	Absent thyroid	Enzyme deficiency
Natural history known	Learning difficulties	Learning difficulties
	Growth failure	Seizures
Safe, acceptable test	Blood spot at 7 days of age	Blood spot at 7 days of age
Sensitive test	Positive when disease present	Positive when disease present
Specific test	Negative when disease not present	Negative when disease not present
Recognized treatment	Thyroxine	Low phenylalanine diet
Benefit from diagnosis	Near normal growth and development	Near normal growth and development

Table 22.1 Criteria for a good screening test: two examples.

lalanine diet results in good outcome. Life-long dietary restriction is recommended. In women with PKU, high phenylalanine levels allow the amino acid to cross the placenta, which may lead to fetal brain damage. In pregnancy, tight dietary control is mandatory.

Galactosaemia

A deficiency of the enzyme (galactose-1-phosphate uridyl transferase) leads to accumulation of galactose. Affected babies become ill almost as soon as they begin to drink milk. Typical presenting features in the first weeks of life include vomiting, weight loss, jaundice and severe infection. The infants have a low blood sugar and may have cataracts. If the diagnosis is considered, the enzyme level is easily measured and successful outcome follows exclusion of lactose (galactose + glucose) from the diet. A lactose-free milk is given.

OSCE Station: Examination of the neck

Clinical approach:

Check
• colour
• anaemia

Inspection
• site
• skin, scars
• swelling
• position of head

Palpation
• position of trachea
• swellings, masses
  ◇ anterior triangles
  ◇ posterior triangles
  ◇ suboccipital

If lymph nodes, consider:
• size of nodes
• are they mobile?
• tenderness, signs of inflammation
• local infection (skin, scalp etc.)
• ENT examination (tonsils, otitis externa)
• generalized lymphadenopathy
• hepatosplenomegaly

If thyroid swelling, consider:
• size and shape (?symmetry)
• smooth/nodular
• ask child to sip and swallow a drink
• thyroid function
  ◇ growth and development
  ◇ facial appearance
  ◇ clinical signs of hypo- or hyperthyroidism

Natalie is 13 years old. Please examine her neck

• pleasant, chatty girl
• early pubertal development

• thyroid swelling
  ◇ smooth
  ◇ non tender
  ◇ symmetrical
  ◇ moves with swallowing
  ◇ no bruit

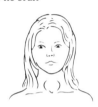

• no other abnormal findings
  ◇ no exophthalmos
  ◇ no tremor of outstretched hands

> Natalie has a goitre.
> She is clinically euthyroid

Never forget:

• say hello and introduce yourself
• general health—is the child ill?
• quickly assess growth, nutrition, and development
• mention the obvious (e.g. drip, tracheostomy)

Look around for:

• medication
• growth measurements

Special points

• examine her neck gently, it can be uncomfortable
• most children have palpable cervical nodes
• lymph nodes are rarely malignant or tuberculous
• goitres
  ◇ commonly auto-immune thyroiditis
  ◇ usually euthyroid, or hypothyroid
  ◇ the cardinal feature of hypo-thyroidism is loss of height velocity
  ◇ classic signs of hypo- or hyper-thyroidism are unusual and appear late in thyroid disease

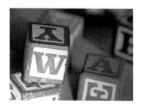

Immunization and Infections

Most illness in childhood is infective, and an important activity in the early life of every individual is meeting and establishing immunity to a wide variety of infecting organisms. Immunological mechanisms in childhood are essentially the same as in adults but are not fully developed at birth. Cellular immunity is effective from birth: for the first 2 or 3 years of life total white cell count is relatively high, lymphocytes predominate over polymorphs in the circulating blood. Pus can be formed at any age. Humoral immunity is slower to develop.

Maternal IgG is transferred across the placenta from early fetal life, giving the full-term infant passive immunity to many infections, including measles, rubella and mumps. In contrast, the larger molecules of IgM do not cross the placenta and the neonate is therefore fully susceptible to some bacterial infections including pertussis. The fetus is capable of mounting its own IgM in response to intrauterine infection, e.g. rubella, but synthesis of other immunoglobulins gets off to a rather sluggish start after birth. Total immunoglobulin levels in all infants are at their lowest at about 3–4 months of age which is another suscep-tible period. A reasonable level of humoral immunity is established by the age of 6–9 months (Fig. 23.1).

Recurrent infections are seldom due to immunological deficiences, although it is important to consider this possibility. Rarely, however, repeated infections may be due to some defect of the cellular or humoral defence mechanisms.

INCREASED SUSCEPTIBILITY TO INFECTION

- Preterm infants
- Socioeconomic deprivation
- Chronic/debilitating illness, e.g. cystic fibrosis, e.g. chronic renal failure
- Immunodeficiency primary or secondary, e.g. treatment of malignancy
- Congenital abnormality, e.g. urinary tract anomalies

Immunization

As infectious diseases account for a large part of the mortality and morbidity of early

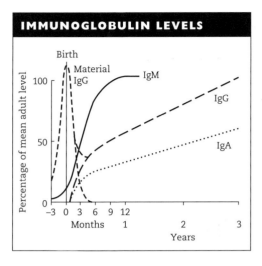

IMMUNOGLOBULIN LEVELS

Fig. 23.1 Immunoglobulin levels in early life.

childhood, it is imperative to make the maximum use of all available preventive measures. All doctors responsible for children must impress on parents the necessity for full immunization, and must themselves be committed to pursuing such a policy with enthusiasm. It is every child's right to be protected against infectious diseases. Widespread immunization in the community increases *herd immunity*, which reduces the chances of transmission of infection between children, and may even allow disease eradication (e.g. smallpox). No child should be denied immunization without serious thought as to the consequences, both for the individual child and for the community.

> Almost 2 million children die each year as a result of disease which can be prevented by vaccination and over 90 000 fall victim to paralytic polio.

In determining such a schedule, two basic decisions are made:
• Against what diseases should a child be protected? This requires a balance of the probabilities of him catching it, suffering death or disability from it and the dangers

and effectiveness of the immunizing procedure. The more common and the more dangerous the disease, and the safer the immunization, the greater the need.
• At what age should immunization be done? This depends upon the age at which the child is susceptible, and the age at which he can best respond to the vaccine. There is often a conflict here, as in the case of pertussis. The greatest danger of the disease is in the first 6 months of life, but the immunological response is relatively poor before 3 months of age (Table 23.1).

Immunization against meningococcal group C infection was commenced in the UK in 1999, starting with infants and students (Table 23.2).

Contraindications

Immunizing procedures should be avoided in children who are acutely unwell. Live vaccines should not be given to those who are immunologically depressed (from disease or drugs), or during pregnancy. Since live vaccine viruses may be transmitted within a household, the risk to a person in that home who is pregnant or is immunosuppressed should be remembered.

UK IMMUNIZATION

Birth	BCG for high-risk groups, e.g. immigrant families
2 months	Polio + Hib/DTP + MenC
3 months	Polio + Hib/DTP + MenC
4 months	Polio + Hib/DTP + MenC
12–15 months	MMR
3–5 years	Polio + DT + MMR
10–14 years	BCG
13–18 years	Polio + DT

Table 23.1 UK immunization schedule. Details and contraindications are in 'The Green Book'—*Immunisation against Infectious Disease* (HMSO).

THE VACCINES

	Protection	Nature	Live	Route
Polio (OPV)	Poliomyelitis	Attenuated virus	Yes*	Oral
Hib	*Haemophilus influenzae* B	Conjugated capsular antigen	No	Intramuscular or deep subcutaneous
DTP	Diphtheria, tetanus, pertussis	Toxoid and bacterial antigen	No	Intramuscular or deep subcutaneous
Men C	Meningococcus group C	Conjugated antigen	No	Intramuscular or deep subcutaneous
MMR	Measles, mumps, rubella	Attenuated viruses	Yes	Intramuscular or deep subcutaneous
BCG	Tuberculosis	Attenuated mycobacterium	Yes	Intradermal

* An inactivated polio vaccine given by SC injection is available for the immunosuppressed child.
BCG, bacille Calmette–Guérin (tuberculosis).

Table 23.2 The vaccines.

Apart from a major reaction to a previous dose of vaccine, there are few other contraindications. *Extreme* hypersensitivity to antibiotics is a contraindication to polio (penicillin, streptomycin, neomycin or polymyxin) and measles (neomycin or kanamycin). Previous anaphylaxis to egg contraindicates MMR. A history of seizures (fits) or eczema is *not* a contraindication.

Unwanted effects

Minor reactions to the pertussis component of Hib/DTP are common—restlessness, fever and crying a few hours after the injection, together with a sore injection site. If that has occurred after the first injection, it is sensible to give paracetamol after subsequent doses.

BCG is injected *intradermally* over the insertion of the deltoid muscle. After 3–6 weeks there is local erythema, induration and sometimes ulceration. The axillary glands may be large and painful. The local signs go in 2–6 months. In school children BCG is given routinely only if the prior tuberculin skin test was negative.

Diagnosis of infections

In children with unexplained fever and in some in whom a firm 'disease diagnosis' has been made (e.g. meningitis), it is important to try to establish the responsible organism.

Infection is found by:

- Identification of the organism
  - By microscopy
  - By culture

- A rise of specific antibody titre

Swabs should be taken thoroughly (especially throat swabs) and transported to the laboratory swiftly. Take all necessary bacteriological specimens before giving antibiotics, if possible. Material for virological culture must be put straight into transport medium. Immunofluorescent techniques allow rapid, positive viral identification, e.g. rotavirus in stool, RSV in nasal secretions. Skin scrapings are needed to identify skin fungi.

Demonstration of a significant rise in antibody titre, whether bacterial (e.g. ASO) or viral, requires at least two specimens, one taken early in the illness, another 10 days to 3 weeks later. A single convalescent sample showing a high antibody titre must be interpreted more cautiously.

Proof of some infections (e.g. HIV, Hepatitis B, meningococcus and pertussis) may be possible by polymerase chain reaction (PCR) tests which detect the relevant DNA material, and provide a rapid result.

Specific fevers

The main clinical features of the important contagious diseases of childhood together with their incubation periods and complications are listed in the table. Infectivity is usually maximal in the prodromal stage and ends within a week of definitive signs appearing. The following paragraphs describe the aspects of these diseases which are important in childhood (Table 23.3).

Measles (morbilli)

This usually presents with respiratory catarrh, misery and fever. About the 4th day a red, maculopapular rash starts behind the ears and spreads to the trunk: less frequent presentations include febrile convulsion and epistaxis. Koplik's spots are small (pinhead) whitish spots on the mucosa inside the cheeks and lower lip. Otitis media and bronchopneumonia are common complications: encephalitis is rare but serious. In the absence of complications, antibiotics are not indicated.

Rubella (German measles)

Rubella may present with rash, respiratory catarrh, or epistaxis. In general, the illness is very mild and there are virtually no complications in childhood. The rash, mainly on the trunk, usually consists of small, pink macules but may be confluent and resemble scarlet fever. The suboccipital lymph glands are usually enlarged. The arthralgia of the hands, so common in adolescent and adult females, does not affect children.

Chickenpox (varicella)

This is usually a mild disease. The differential diagnosis is from papular urticaria (p. 185) which, if scratched and infected, also presents papules, vesicles, pustules and scabs. However, the lesions in chickenpox are predominantly on the trunk, whilst papular urticaria is peripherally distributed.

CONTAGIOUS DISEASES

Disease	Incubation period (days)*	Main features	Important complications	Laboratory findings
Measles	7-10-12	Misery, fever, catarrh, cough, conjunctivitis; Koplik's spots, blotchy, red rash on face and trunk	Pneumonia Otitis media Encephalitis	Rise in antibody titre Immunofluorescence of naso-pharyngeal aspirate
Rubella	10-18-21	Upper respiratory catarrh; macular or erythematous rash; chiefly on trunk, cervical adenopathy	Virtually none in childhood. Encephalitis very rare	Virus culture from stool or nose Rise in antibody titre
Chickenpox	10-14-21	Rash on trunk, perineum and, scalp: papules, vesicles pustules, scabs: fever at pustular stage	Conjunctival lesions Encephalitis	EM of vesicular fluid Virus culture Monoclonal antibody
Mumps	14-18-28	Parotitis, sometimes involvement of other salivary glands	Meningitis Pancreatitis Orchitis after puberty	Virus from saliva Rise in antibody titre Lymphocytosis
Whooping cough	7-10-14	Upper respiratory catarrh: paroxysmal cough with vomiting. Modified greatly by immunization	Pneumonia Lobar collapse Convulsions Haemorrhage (nose, eyes, brain)	B. pertussis from per nasal swab. Immunofluorescence Lymphocytosis +++ PCR test
Scarlet fever	1-3-7	Tonsillitis (pharyngitis); diffuse, erythematous rash chiefly on trunk; sore, coated tongue: circumoral pallor	Otitis media Rheumatic fever Acute nephritis	Group A haem Strep, from throat Rise in ASO titre

* Outer figures, range; central figure, usual. PCR, polymerase chain reaction.

Table 23.3 Contagious diseases.

Complications are rare. Chickenpox encephalitis presents as ataxia a week or so after the rash has appeared: the prognosis is good.

Mumps

This is most commonly confused with cervical adenitis. The exact location of the swelling, the fact that it is nearly always bilateral, the swelling of the orifice of the parotid ducts, and absence of any cause for cervical adenitis, should make the diagnosis clear. Mumps meningitis can occur without parotitis. Rarely nerve deafness occurs, usually unilateral. Pancreatitis and orchitis are rare before puberty.

Whooping cough (pertussis)

Whooping cough is a bacterial infection caused by *Bordetella pertussis*. It is a serious disease in the very young infant, and unpleasant at all ages. Babies with pertussis do not whoop, but the cough is paroxysmal and associated with vomiting. Infants may present with an apnoea attack, a day or two before the cough develops. Severe spasms may lead to capillary rupture (which is common in the conjunctivae) or may lead to hypoxia sufficient to cause a seizure. Lobar collapse is not uncommon.

In children who have been immunized, the disease tends to be mild, the whoop absent, and there may be no lymphocytosis; the diagnosis is then easily missed.

EXCLUSION FROM NURSERY/SCHOOL

Parents are advised to allow their child, once well, to return to school:
• 5 days after appearance of rash for chickenpox and rubella
• 5 days after starting antibiotics for whooping cough.

Roseola infantum (exanthem subitum)

Roseola infantum, caused by Herpes virus 6 and 7, is a mild disease of infants and young children, and rarely severe enough to need admission. Catarrhal symptoms and fever for 3 or 4 days are followed by the abrupt appearance of light red, discrete macules on the trunk. As the rash appears, the fever rapidly settles and the child is greatly improved. A few days later, the illness is over.

Erythema infectiosum (Fifth disease/slapped cheek disease)

This mildly contagious disease is caused by a human parvovirus. It commences on the face with bright red cheeks ('slapped face'). Subsequently maculopapular red spots appear on the limbs with a symmetrical distribution beginning on the extensor surfaces and spreading to the flexor surfaces and then to the buttocks and trunk. The rash subsides over the course of a week but may recur in response to a variety of skin irritants. Aplastic crises are an important complication in children with a chronic haemolytic anaemia.

Infectious mononucleosis (glandular fever)

Glandular fever results from infection with Epstein–Barr virus (Herpes virus 4), but a similar clinical picture may result from infection by *cytomegalovirus* or *Toxoplasma gondii*.

The presentation is variable: the onset may be gradual with malaise, anorexia and low-grade fever for one to two weeks, or it may begin abruptly with high fever and headache. Specific signs include:
• pharyngitis, often exudative and oedematous
• lymphadenopathy—multiple, firm, discrete, non-tender glands especially in the neck

- hepato-splenomegaly and hepatitis
- rash, macular or urticarial. Ampicillin or amoxycillin causes a florid rash
- meningeal involvement, with headache, stiff neck, and raised cells and protein in the CSF.

In classic glandular fever, the blood shows an increased number of mononuclear cells (lymphocytes and monocytes) with atypical lymphocytes ('glandular fever cells'). There may be thrombocytopenia. The Paul-Bunnell (heterophil antibody) test is positive after the first week or two of illness. In practice, a simplified version of this test (Monospot) is generally used. Specific EBV serology is more reliable.

Hepatitis A (infectious hepatitis)

Worldwide, this is the commonest cause of childhood jaundice. It is seen most frequently where hygiene is poor. It is milder in children than in adults.

HEPATITIS A

Prodrome (week 1)

- Anorexia, malaise

- Nausea/abdominal pain

Jaundice (weeks 2–3)

- Tender hepatomegaly

- Pale stools, dark urine

- Urine urobilinogen ↑ and bile ↑

- Serum
  - Bilirubin ↑
  - Liver enzymes (AST, ALT) ↑

Differential diagnosis in the preicteric and non-icteric cases is from other causes of abdominal pain and vomiting. Once jaundice has developed, diagnosis is not difficult. Urobilinogen may be detected in the pre-icteric stage and may be the sole diagnostic clue in the mildest cases without clinical jaundice. Serum bilirubin is raised, with roughly equal parts conjugated and unconjugated. Complications are rare. Jaundice usually fades in 1–2 weeks but exceptionally persists for months.

Transmission is usually by the faecal–oral route, therefore cross-infection should be prevented as far as possible by good hygiene. However, infectivity is greatest before jaundice appears and it is quite common to have more than one case in a household.

In the average case the child will be in bed for a few days and kept off school for 2–3 weeks.

Herpes

HSV Type I infections are very common: and usually asymptomatic. Spread is by infected saliva: primary infection involves the mouth, skin or eye.

HSV Type II is a genital infection of importance in the newborn baby, and in children incurring sexual abuse.

Herpetic stomatitis results from a primary infection with HSV I, and is most common in toddlers. There are vesicles, ulcers and scabs on the lips and tongue, the gums are inflamed and the child drools. There is cervical adenitis. Because of pain, the child may not eat or drink and admission to hospital may be necessary to maintain fluid intake. The condition is self-limiting, the discomfort easing after a few days; the lesions have healed within two weeks. Reactivation of herpes simplex infection commonly presents as a *cold sore* on the lip, tending to recur at times of infection, exposure to sunshine or other stress. Someone with gingivostomatitis or a cold sore may easily auto-inoculate themselves, or another person, causing a herpetic whitlow of the finger, eye infection (keratoconjunctivitis) or vulvo vaginitis.

People with cold sores should not kiss children.

Herpes encephalitis may occur during primary infection, or reactivation of the virus, and in the absence of other features of herpes infection. It is a severe encephalopathy with a high morbidity and mortality despite treatment with aciclovir.

Enteroviruses

Coxsackie and echo viruses are common causes of brief febrile illnesses associated with respiratory and gastrointestinal symptoms. Faecal oral transmission is usual, and outbreaks are most common in the autumn. Some are associated with ulcers confined to the posterior pharynx— *herpangina*. In addition to mouth ulcers, some coxsackie A group viruses are associated with vesicles on the hands, feet and buttocks —*hand, foot and mouth disease.*

Complications from enteroviral infection are rare in healthy children.

Meningococcal disease

The gram-negative diplococcus *(Neisseria meningitidis)* (meningococcus) is divided into several sero-groups: groups B and C are most prevalent in the UK.

Meningococcal disease is an important cause of morbidity in the UK (nearly 2000 cases per year) and a case fatality rate of just over 10%. Transmission is via close contact with nasopharyngeal droplets. Infections are commoner in winter.

The peak incidence is at 6–8 months of age, with a smaller second peak in teenagers (of whom 25% are nasopharyngeal carriers). The incubation period is 2–10 days.

The presentation varies according to the dominance of either septicaemia or meningitis.

MENINGOCOCCAL INFECTION

- 25% septicaemia
- 60% septicaemia and meningitis
- 15% meningitis alone.

Septicaemia

Mild non-specific symptoms are followed within days, or within hours (in severe cases), by severe illness and fever and the rapid appearance of a widespread red macular rash which soon becomes purpuric (not blanching on pressure). The rash may be sparse or profuse, and may vary from tiny petechial spots to large purpuric lesions which coalesce to form large ecchymoses. Septic shock follows in 30% of cases and requires prompt diagnosis and treatment. Severely ill children require treatment in a paediatric intensive care unit, others can be treated safely with antibiotics, plasma expanders and antipyretics on the children's ward.

> **i** A feverish ill child who has a purpuric rash should be given benzylpenicillin IV or IM and then transferred to hospital

Meningococcus may be grown from pharyngeal swab, blood culture, aspirate of skin lesions or CSF. PCR tests provide confirmation of diagnosis.

There is an increased risk of disease in the child's close contacts at home or in the nursery, though such secondary cases are rare. Close contacts are given a 2-day course of rifampicin (as is the affected child before leaving hospital) to lessen the risk of such secondary infection. They should be warned that rifampicin makes their urine pink.

A young child may be well in the morning and dead in the evening as a result of meningococcal septicaemia.

Meningococcus is the commonest cause of bacterial meningitis in Europe. (Features are described on p. 108.)

Children are now immunized against group C meningococcus, but not for group B.

Kawasaki disease

This is a rare but important disease. It presents as a systemic febrile vasculitis affecting children under the age of 5. No causative organism has been identified. It is the commonest cause of acquired heart disease in childhood in developed countries (where rheumatic fever is rare). Coronary arteritis leads to the formation of aneurysms in up to 30% of children.

Apart from the classical presentations, there may be other systemic features which dominate and lead to delays in diagnosis, and therefore the duration of high fever for more than 5 days is a particularly helpful sign. A useful occasional sign is redness and induration at the site of a previous BCG scar.

Providing that the diagnosis is made early, intravenous immunoglobulin given within 10 days of illness onset decreases the incidence and severity of coronary aneurysms.

DIAGNOSTIC CRITERIA FOR KAWASAKI DISEASE

At least five of the following six:
- Fever >5 days
- Inflamed mouth, cracked lips, red pharynx
- Bilateral conjunctivitis
- Polymorphous rash
- Hand/foot reddening, oedema and later desquamation
- Cervical lymphadenopathy >15 mm, unilateral non-purulent

Tuberculosis

Tuberculosis is common wherever poverty, malnutrition and overcrowding are prevalent, and rare where standards of hygiene and nutrition are good. In the developing countries of the world, tuberculosis appears in forms that were common in Europe 50 years ago. TB is rampaging through the African population along with HIV. The chief sources of infection are adults with sputum-positive pulmonary tuberculosis (Mycobacterium tuberculosis), and milk from infected cattle (Mycobacterium bovis). Prevention depends first upon general improvement in socioeconomic conditions, and second upon specific measures including the prompt recognition and treatment of infectious adults, BCG immunization, tuberculin testing of cattle and pasteurization of milk.

The initial infection is in the lungs if conveyed by droplets, in the bowel if conveyed by milk. The first site of infection is known as the primary focus. The primary complex comprises the primary focus and the enlarged lymph nodes draining it. Spread of infection beyond the local nodes may result in tubercle bacilli reaching the blood stream, causing either tuberculous septicaemia (miliary TB) or infection of distant organs (meninges, kidneys, bones and joints). Tuberculous cervical lymph nodes are thought to be infected via the tonsils. Erythema nodosum may be caused by tuberculosis (p. 185).

In the UK, childhood tuberculosis is uncommon. Primary complexes in the lung are seen more often in immigrant children from Asia than in others. Tuberculous meningitis is a rare disease of great importance.

> [i] The WHO estimates an annual incidence of over 8 million cases of TB in the world, 95% of them live in developing countries.
> The WHO Global Tuberculosis Control Programme now reaches half of the world population.

Pulmonary tuberculosis

The child with a primary complex has minimal symptoms. Haemoptysis and systemic symptoms are exceptional. Children with TB, traced through their contact with infected adults, are often symptom-free. Diagnosis is based on the X-ray appearances and a positive tuberculin test. Sputum is not usually present, but tubercle bacilli may be recovered from gastric washings.

> [i] Three million of the world's population die from TB each year.

Tuberculous meningitis

> A child with a lymphocytic meningitis, and low CSF glucose, should be treated for TB until proved otherwise.

This disease, which was universally fatal before the discovery of streptomycin, is still a serious disease, especially in infancy. It most commonly affects young children; the onset is insidious so that there is usually a history of weight loss or poor weight gain, vague malaise, anorexia and perhaps slight fever. After a few days, evidence of meningeal involvement is shown by headache, drowsiness, irritability and neck stiffness. If the diagnosis is not made at this stage, convulsions, focal signs and impairment of consciousness supervene. The clinical signs are those of meningitis (p. 108). The CSF has a raised lymphocyte count, with raised protein and low glucose.

Cervical adenopathy

Tuberculous neck glands are rare in the UK. Usually a single gland or group of glands is affected, on one side of the neck. The gland is firm (unless caseating), partially fixed and not especially tender. In contrast, cervical glands with recurrent tonsillitis are usually bilateral, fairly soft and mobile, and only rarely form a localized abscess requiring drainage. In TB, the tuberculin test is positive.

CERVICAL LYMPHADENOPATHY

Differential diagnosis
- Reactive (e.g. tonsillitis)
- TB
- Malignancy (lymphoma, leukaemia)
- Other infections (e.g. glandular fever, rubella, atypical mycobacteria, toxoplasma).

Management

Regardless of the site, the management of tuberculosis can be divided into three parts.

- **Notification** of the case so that contacts can be immunized and possible sources of infection identified.
- **Antituberculous drugs**: rifampicin, pyrazinamide and isoniazid form the basis of treatment. Treatment should be continued for at least 6 months.
- **General management**: Children should not be admitted to hospital or kept off school without good reason. A pulmonary primary complex is rarely infectious, and isolation is unnecessary. If nutrition is unsatisfactory, it should be improved.

HIV

Worldwide, by the year 2000, over 4 million children had died of AIDS, 1.5 million were known to be infected, and 13 million had become orphans because of the disease. In children HIV Type I is usual, and in developed countries vertical transmission from mother to child is the usual route of infection. Infection from blood products still occurs in developing countries.

Infected babies appear normal at birth, but without prophylaxis nearly 25%

develop AIDS or die in the first year. The rest show a much slower disease progression with some showing no evidence of indicator diseases until the teenage years.

AIDS INDICATOR DISEASES

- Opportunist infection
- Recurrent bacterial infections
- Failure to thrive
- Encephalopathy
- Malignancy.

The HIV antibody test is unreliable in infancy because of maternal antibody transmission. Children over 18 months who have HIV antibody are infected. PCR tests are increasingly used for diagnosis. Prophylactic treatment is begun as soon as HIV infection is suspected, and some units give prophylaxis to all children born to HIV positive mothers from birth. Vertical transmission is reduced to <10% if mother is given antiretroviral therapy in pregnancy, delivery is by caesarian section, and breast feeding is avoided.

Malaria

Malaria is endemic in many parts of the world and may be seen in immigrants from malarious areas or in persons who have visited such places within the preceding 4 months. It usually presents with fever which does not necessarily show the classic periodic pattern. The spleen may be enlarged. Diagnosis depends on identification of parasites in blood smears, and may be easier *between* peaks of fever. It may be necessary to examine several smears.

Plasmodium can develop resistance to drugs. The appropriate treatment varies according to the local sensitivity of the responsible organism. Prophylactic drugs must be taken throughout residence in a

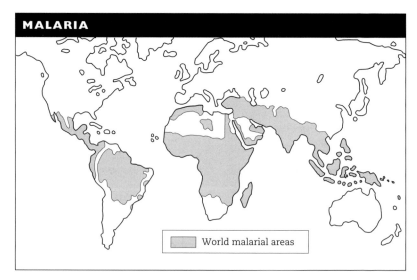

Fig. 23.2 Distribution of malarial endemic areas.

NOTIFIABLE DISEASES

Diphtheria	Mumps
Dysentery	Paratyphoid
Encephalitis	Poliomyelitis
Food poisoning	Rubella
Hepatitis A and B	Scarlet fever
Measles	Tetanus
Malaria	Tuberculosis
Meningitis	Typhoid
Meningococcal	Whooping cough
septicaemia	

Table 23.4 Notification of infectious diseases.

malarial area *and for at least 4 weeks thereafter* (Fig. 23.2).

Notification of infectious diseases

Doctors are required, for public health and epidemiological reasons, to notify to the Consultant in Communicable Disease Control, or the Director of Public Health a number of infectious diseases (Table 23.4).

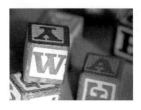

Accidents and Non-accidents

Accidents are the commonest cause of death in children over the age of 1 year (p. 3). In England and Wales, nearly 500 children die each year; 65% are boys. Road traffic accidents involve mainly children of school age, accidents in the home involve mainly children under the age of five. By the age of 11, one in four children has experienced a serious accident.

The risk of accident is influenced by social circumstances. The child in a large family in poor housing, on the street much of the day and ostensibly supervised by another child only marginally older, is at great hazard; and the mother trying to care for young children at the top of a tower block, without the privilege of an enclosed garden or play space, has a difficult task. Pedestrian accidents are commonest in the 5–9 age group when parents are falsely confident about their child's skills: it is wiser to under-estimate, rather than over-estimate a child's abilities. In general, children cannot cross a busy road safely, even at a traffic light, on their own until the age of 8 or 9 years, and cannot ride a bicycle safely on a main road until 13.

There is great need for better education of children and parents about safety, and for legislation to minimize the opportunities for accidents.

> **Government objective:**
> To reduce the death rate for accidents amongst children to less than 4.5 per 100 000 by the year 2005.

Head injury

Initial treatment concentrates on the child's Airways, Breathing and Circulation. Subsequent management of head injuries calls for some experience. On the one hand, scalps split easily and bleed profusely, but the quantity of blood may cause unjustifiable alarm. On the other hand, some apparently trivial injuries are associated with intracranial bleeding that only becomes apparent after an interval of time. A linear skull fracture without displacement may be unimportant, whilst intracranial bleeding may occur without a fracture. If in doubt, admit the child for 24 hours and observe. Record pulse, respiratory rate, blood pressure, level of consciousness and pupillary size and reactions (Fig. 24.2).

Burns and scalds

Scalds are caused by hot fluids and cause predominantly loss of the epidermis only, with blistering and peeling. However, the

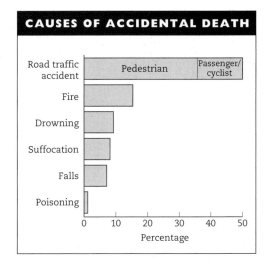

Fig. 24.1 Causes of accidental death.

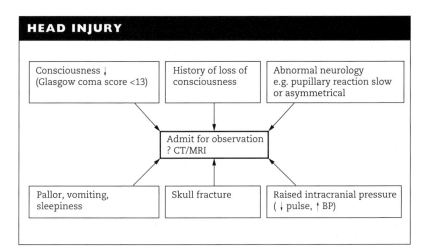

Fig. 24.2 Management of head injury.

skin of young children sometimes suffers full thickness loss from comparatively minor scalds. There is a strong argument for limiting the maximum temperature of hot water in the home to 54°C (129°F). Most scalds occur in the kitchen: parents should be advised to use electric kettles with short coiled flexes which reduce the risk of a child reaching up and pulling the kettle over.

Burns are caused by direct contact with very hot objects or by the clothes catching fire, and result in full thickness skin loss. Loss of skin surface leads to loss of fluid and shock (Fig. 24.3). If more than 10% of the body surface is involved, intravenous fluid therapy will be required. Burns involving 50% or more of the body surface carry a grave prognosis, although children

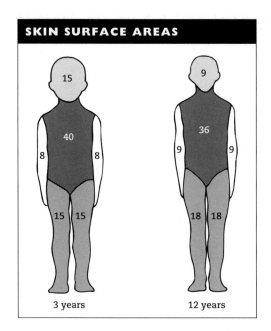

SKIN SURFACE AREAS

3 years

12 years

Fig. 24.3 Skin surface areas at 3 and 12 years. The figures indicate the percentage of total body surface represented by each part.

have survived more extensive burns than this.

As a general rule, burns and scalds are more serious than they seem, and hospital admission is advisable for all but the most trivial.

Poisoning

Accidental poisoning is very common and usually occurs in toddlers aged 2–4 years, who are sufficiently agile to find and swallow things, yet not old enough to appreciate the dangers. The parent finds the 3 year old with an empty bottle in the bathroom or kitchen and is unsure how much the child has ingested. Usually the child has swallowed little or nothing, and it is a poisoning scare rather than a true poisoning event. Less than 15% of the thousands of children presenting to hospital because of accidental poisoning develop symptoms; death is extremely rare.

The things that children swallow are numberless, but fall into three main categories:

• Tablets and medicines: analgesics, sleeping tablets, tranquillizers, antidepressants and iron. They are a more common cause of morbidity than substances in the other two groups below.

• Household and horticultural fluids: bleach, turpentine, paraffin, cleaning fluids and weedkillers.

• Berries and seeds. Laburnum tops the list with deadly nightshade and toadstools featuring commonly. In the UK, things plucked from the hedgerows and ditches hardly ever cause serious illness.

Occasionally younger children are given poisons by their parents (Table 24.1). If older children in the prepubertal-adolescent age range swallow poisonous substances (usually drugs), this is indicative of an emotional upset. Most often it is done as a gesture of defiance, or a wish for temporary oblivion, rather than with serious

POISONING

	Accidental	Self harm	Deliberate (by parent)
Occurrence	Very common	Common	Uncommon
Age (years)	2–4	>10	0–5
Substance	Anything	Analgesic	Prescribed drug
Quantity	Little or nothing	Variable	Large
Recurrence risk	Small	Medium	Large

Table 24.1 Characteristic patterns in different types of poisoning.

intention to commit suicide. Nevertheless, some are pathologically depressed and the advice of a child psychiatrist should be sought when schoolchildren have swallowed poison.

Management

- Identify poison
- Estimate maximum amount/toxicity
- Minimize absorption (? emesis, lavage, charcoal)
- Promote excretion (fluids/purgatives)
- Combat symptoms

If a large amount of a potentially dangerous poison has been ingested in the previous 6 h, the stomach should be emptied.

Emesis usually follows the administration of 20 mL ipecacuanha syrup in orange juice, repeated if necessary. Gastric lavage may be needed if emesis does not occur, or if the child is unconscious.

Do not induce emesis if:
- The child is not fully conscious

- Caustics (bleaches, acids)
  - (↑ Risk of perforation)

- Hydrocarbons (turpentine)
  - (↑ Risk of pneumonitis)

Absorption may be discouraged by diluting the poison (milk is good and usually available), by giving an absorbent agent such as activated charcoal or by giving a specific antidote (e.g. desferrioxamine in iron poisoning). Excretion may be encouraged by the use of purgatives or forced diuresis in selected cases.

It is usually advisable to admit poisoned children to hospital for observation for at least a few hours. The *Regional Drug Information Centres* provide helpful information and advice. (Their telephone numbers are listed in the *British National Formulary*.)

Accident prevention is a major health priority (Fig. 24.4).

Chronic lead poisoning

Lead poisoning is uncommon in the UK. Lead water pipes have been replaced by copper, and drinking water is drawn from main supplies. Modern paints contain very little lead. Nevertheless, some risks still exist: industrial sources (smelting works), disused car batteries (as a fuel) or a history of ingestion of paint/dirt—*pica* (pica is the Latin name for magpie, a bird notorious for stealing and consuming almost anything).

Early symptoms include abdominal colic, pallor, anaemia, irritability, anorexia and disturbed sleep. Later symptoms are predominantly neurological, including encephalopathy, neuropathy and seizures.

RECREATIONAL DRUGS

Name	Street names	Formulation	Undesired effects
Opiates	Scag; smack; dragon; tiger	Methadone: liquid powder wrapped in foil/ prescription opiates	Respiratory depression Coma Pin-point pupils Hypotension
Hallucinogens	Tabs; LSD; acid; trips; magic mushrooms	Small squares of absorbent paper with pattern /microdots (tiny pellets)/ mushrooms	Psychotic symptoms Accidents
Cocaine	Coke; snow; base; crack; wash; rocks	White powder Paper wrapped or twisted	Agitation Dilated pupils Tachycardia Hypertension
Amphetamines	Speed; uppers; sweets; whiz; ecstasy; E's; doves	Powder Tabs Capsules Homemade tabs	Agitation/paranoia Hallucination Hypertension Dehydration Hyperthermia Delirium/coma Convulsions/coma
Cannabis	Pot; dose; grass; ganja; weed; spliff; joint	Resin blocks; dried leaf	Anxiety attacks Panic disorder

Table 24.2 Recreational drugs.

Permanent brain damage may result in learning difficulties.

> **Government objective:**
> To reduce smoking prevalence among 11–15-year-olds to less than 6%.

Recreational drugs

Drugs of abuse are now relatively cheap and widely available. Solvent abuse (inhalation of glues and aerosols) is becoming less prevalent. Tobacco and alcohol should not be overlooked: there is growing concern and awareness of teenage alcoholism and its combination with other agents may be lethal.

Currently the aim is to give children honest, realistic information (Table 24.2). There is no point in pretending to the child who knows how to procure drugs that they harm all who take them. Drugs education in school is seen by some as contentious. Parents may be alerted by finding drug taking equipment or by noticing changes in their child's behaviour. The national drugs

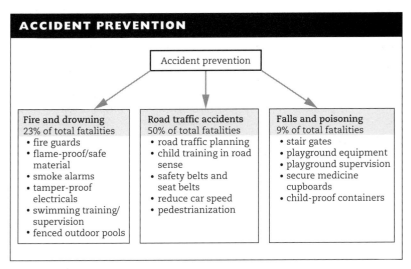

ACCIDENT PREVENTION

Accident prevention

Fire and drowning
23% of total fatalities
- fire guards
- flame-proof/safe material
- smoke alarms
- tamper-proof electricals
- swimming training/ supervision
- fenced outdoor pools

Road traffic accidents
50% of total fatalities
- road traffic planning
- child training in road sense
- safety belts and seat belts
- reduce car speed
- pedestrianization

Falls and poisoning
9% of total fatalities
- stair gates
- playground equipment
- playground supervision
- secure medicine cupboards
- child-proof containers

Fig. 24.4 Accident prevention.

helpline or local organizations are helpful contacts.

In children who become ill after taking such agents, it is important to be aware that adverse effects arise from the drug, contaminants or other agents added to the mixture. Solvents may lead to asphyxia, cardiac dysrhythmias and hepato-renal failure.

Child abuse and neglect

> *Abuse*: deliberately inflicted injury
> *Neglect*: inadequate or negligent parenting, failing to protect the child

Many children suffer a combination of abuse and neglect. The definitions suggest that abuse is an active process and neglect a passive one, but for most forms of abuse the parents, who are the usual perpetrators, contribute to the abuse by both active and passive roles. Thus the spouse who fails to intervene when their partner sexually abuses the child is a passive partner to the abuse and colluding with it. A parent who passively fails to provide food or love may also indulge in active physical assault.

TYPES OF ABUSE

- Physical abuse
- Neglect
- Sexual abuse
- Emotional abuse
- Munchausen syndrome by proxy

A child is considered to be abused if he or she is treated by an adult in a way that is unacceptable in a given culture at a given time. It is important to recognize that children are treated differently not only in different countries but in different subcultures of one city and that there will be various opinions about what constitutes abuse. With the passage of time standards change: corporal punishment is much less acceptable than it was 10 years ago. These factors contribute to the difficulties of determining changes in the prevalence of abuse.

Physical abuse (non-accidental injury)

Such abuse is usually short-term and violent though it may be repetitive. Infants and toddlers are most at risk. Soft tissue injuries to the skin, ears and eyes are common as well as injuries to the joints and bones (Fig. 24.5).

The most common forms of injury are:
• Bruising, especially of the face and trunk. The bruises may be multiple and of different ages. (But remember that a normal active toddler is likely to have five or six bruises of different ages, usually on the shins.)
• Fractures, especially of the ribs, humerus and femur. Fractures at different stages of healing, denoting repetitive injury, or involving an infant are particularly suspicious.
• Head injury, skull fracture and subdural haematoma may occur from direct injury or shaking. Depressed and complicated (as opposed to simple linear) fractures are particularly suspicious. Retinal haemorrhages may occur. The most severe head injuries will cause intraventricular and intracerebral haemorrhage leading to death or permanent brain damage.
• Burns, either from cigarettes or holding a child close to a fire. Scalds, from immersion in very hot water (usually involving a hand, foot or buttock).

Neglect

Failing to provide the love, care, food or physical circumstances that will allow the child to grow and develop normally, or exposing a child to any kind of danger, constitutes neglect.

Neglect and injury are closely associated and both are indications of parental inadequacy. The child may show evidence of poor standards of hygiene or nutrition; height

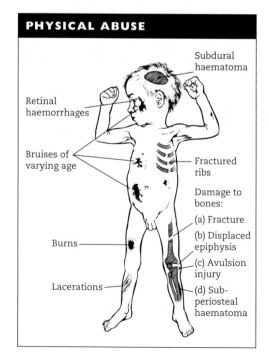

PHYSICAL ABUSE

Subdural haematoma

Retinal haemorrhages

Bruises of varying age

Fractured ribs

Damage to bones:

(a) Fracture

(b) Displaced epiphysis

Burns

(c) Avulsion injury

Lacerations

(d) Sub-periosteal haematoma

Fig. 24.5 Characteristic injuries caused by physical abuse.

Helpful diagnostic features suggesting non-accidental injury

- Delay in seeking medical advice.
- The explanation is incompatible with the injury observed (a baby's skull does not fracture if he rolls off the sofa onto a carpeted floor).
- The story of the accident varies.
- The child is brought to the doctor by someone other than the person in whose presence the injury occurred.
- Unusual parental behaviour with the parents being more interested in their own feelings, and in returning home, than in concern for the child. (Sometimes the parents will leave the child in hospital before the senior doctor has arrived.)
- Abnormal parent–child interaction, with the child looking frightened or withdrawn.

---

and weight, when plotted on a growth record, may be well below the expected centile (*non-organic failure to thrive*). Neglect is often combined with emotional abuse.

Sexual abuse

Child sexual abuse includes any use of children for the sexual gratification of adults. It ranges from inappropriate fondling and masturbation to intercourse and buggery. Children may be forced to appear in pornographic photographs or videos, or participate in sex rings or ritual abuse. *Organized abuse* is the term used to describe abuse involving either a number of children, or a number of abusers.

PRESENTATIONS OF SEXUAL ABUSE

- Local
  - Trauma
  - Infection
  - Perineal soreness
  - Discharge or bleeding

- Behaviour change
  - Anorexia
  - Encopresis
  - Self harm

- Sexual behaviour inappropriate for the child's age or environment

Children of all ages, and either sex, are abused, though the commonest is for a girl to be abused by a male who is either a relative or a member of the household.

Emotional abuse (psychological abuse)

Emotional abuse occurs whenever the child receives the repeated message that he or she is worthless, unloved, or unwanted (or only of use in meeting the parents' needs). It ranges from the failure of parents to provide consistent love to overt hostility including spurning, terrorizing, isolating, corrupting and exploiting, or merely denying the child the right to emotional responsiveness. For an infant this may result in failure to thrive with recurrent minor infections and frequent attendances at hospitals and health centres, general developmental delay, and a lack of social responsiveness. The older child is likely to be short, developmentally immature and with delayed language skills. His or her behaviour is likely to be over-active, impulsive and aggressive.

All abuse entails some emotional ill-treatment but currently it is uncommon for emotional abuse alone to be the sole reason for child protection measures through legal action, even though its consequences can be more severe than occasional episodes of physical abuse.

Munchausen syndrome by proxy (MSbP)

This term encompasses a range of behaviour, usually by mothers, in which false illness is invented (for the child) for personal gain. It commonly includes both physical and emotional abuse. The harmful behaviour lies at the far end of the spectrum of inappropriate ways in which parents may behave in relation to childhood illness.

MSbP: SPECTRUM OF BEHAVIOUR

In order of increasing severity

- Anxious parents
  ⇒ Perceives symptoms or signs

- Doctor shopping
  ⇒ Seeking repetitive consultation and investigation

- Enforced invalidism
  ⇒ Increased disability and incapacity when a genuine problem is present

- Fabricated illness (MSbP)
  ⇒ False story and fabricated signs
  ⇒ Altered health record
  ⇒ Direct injury, e.g. poisoning, smothering

The consequences for the child in terms of unpleasant and harmful investigations and treatments, the induction of genuine disease, and the effects of poisoning or suffocation can be disastrous. Furthermore, the child may be encouraged to be a chronic invalid and believe himself to be disabled and unable to attend school and may develop somatoform or factitious behaviour (e.g. Munchausen syndrome) as an adult.

Prevalence of child abuse and neglect

Four per cent of children up to the age of 12 are notified to social service departments because of suspected abuse. Some of that abuse may be mild but at least 1 child per 1000 under the age of 4 suffers severe physical abuse, e.g. fractures, brain haemorrhage or mutilation. This week at least four children in the UK will die as a result of abuse or neglect.

There is some evidence that there may have been an increase in child abuse in the past 5 years, but the apparent increase may be more the result of greater unwillingness by society to tolerate child abuse, increased public awareness and professional recognition.

Perpetrators

Most child abuse occurs in the home and the parents are the usual abusers. Physical abuse, emotional abuse and neglect are often inflicted by both parents. Sex abuse is more common by fathers; poisoning, smothering and MSbP by the mother.

Abuse occurs in all sections of society, but probably occurs more commonly in poor families — 'Destructiveness is the outcome of unlived life'.

Abused deprived children are more likely to become abusing, neglecting parents — the cycle of deprivation.

The motives for abuse are complex. We can all understand how a weary parent in an overcrowded home, where the children are on top of one another, and the father is on shift work attempting to sleep, hits out impatiently at a fractious overdemanding child. However, much abuse is repetitive and, seemingly, premeditated. Often it is an expression of the parent's inner violence and their wish to exert power over their child. It is common for normal parents to have mixed feelings about their children and to have moments when they hate their child. Most parents can control their feelings but a minority injure their child during those feelings of hatred. They are not suffering mental illness but they do have a personality disorder.

Management of child abuse and neglect

All doctors should have a low threshold for suspecting abuse and be prepared to refer the child for more detailed assessment.

> In suspected abuse:
> * Record history carefully (and who provided it).
> * Sketch injuries
> * Photograph
> * Skeletal survey
> * Check Child Protection Register

If abuse is likely the doctor (or other concerned person) will contact the Social Services Department who usually convene a case conference (Fig. 24.6). The aim is to form a clear picture of the child and family relationships and then, making the child's interests paramount, recommendations are made for the child's future safety, including decisions about future legal proceedings. If the child is in imminent danger an *Emergency Protection Order* may be sought from a magistrate. This allows the child to be detained in a hospital or foster home whilst enquiries are made. In view of the high incidence of abuse in siblings, it is

> Information may be obtained and discussion may be necessary with the following:
> * Child
> * GP
> * Parents
> * Health visitor
> * Family
> * Hospital staff
> * Neighbours
> * Social services school/nursery
> * Police

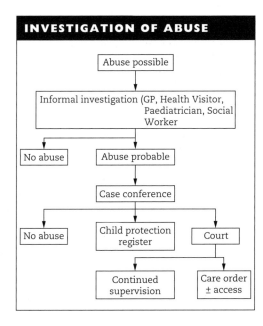

Fig. 24.6 The usual course of investigation of alleged child abuse.

mandatory to check the other children in the child's home.

Subsequent court action may be needed to take a child into the care of the local authority if the risk of further abuse at home is too great (p. 8). More commonly the child is placed on the *Child Protection Register* and skilled help arranged for the families so that the child can be supervised at home and the family helped to modify their behaviour. This help and supervision is normally provided by local authority social workers or the *National Society for the Prevention of Cruelty to Children (NSPCC)*. Further abuse occurs in up to 20% of cases; the recurrence rate is a sensitive index of the effectiveness of management.

The police are represented at case conferences and may be asked to investigate more serious or difficult cases. Only a minority of cases end with a criminal prosecution.

Sudden infant death syndrome (SIDS, cot death)

The sudden death of an infant which is unexpected by history, and in which a thorough post mortem examination fails to demonstrate an adequate cause, occurs in 1 per 1500 live births. In the UK, cot death constitutes about one-fifth of infant deaths.

Most occur at home between the ages of 4 weeks and 4 months, in urban rather than rural areas, during the night, in homes which are socially and economically deprived. The infants' mothers tend to be younger and to smoke.

SIDS is a categorization rather than an explanation. It is a label of exclusion. Many hypotheses have been proposed to explain SIDS: it is likely that there are several differ-

PREVENTION OF SIDS

- **Back to sleep**
  - avoid sleeping prone

- **Not too hot, light bed clothes**
  - 16–20°C overnight, head exposed, no hat

- **Feet to foot**
  - Baby's feet touching foot of cot

- **Smoke free zone**
  - Avoid smoking in pregnancy and in the home

- **Prompt medical advice**
  - If unwell, feverish, or less responsive

ent causes. Hyperthermia or overheating is an important factor, and is the reason for some of the preventative measures. A hundred years ago it was customary to attribute most cot deaths to 'overlaying' (*smothering*) by the mother, whether accidental or deliberate. The proportion of SIDS deaths caused by parents today is likely to be over 10%, and becomes relatively larger and more important as natural causes diminish. Features suggesting an unnatural cause include: previous episodes of apnoea or unexplained illness, recent discharge from hospital, or previous unexpected childhood death in the family.

Sudden unexpected death causes a profound family crisis and the bereaved parents need expert counselling and help. Commonly such parents are invited to enrol in the CONI (Care of Next Infant) programme when they have a subsequent baby. Many are lent an apnoea alarm; though this may be reassuring, evidence is lacking that the alarms prevent cot death.

Appendices

Measurement and conversion

To metric

1 ounce	=	28.4 grams (g)
1 pound	=	0.45 kilogram (kg)
1 fluid ounce	=	28.4 millilitres (mL)
1 pint	=	0.56 litre (L)
1 inch	=	2.54 centimetres (cm)

From metric

1 kilogram	=	2.2 pounds (lb)
1 litre	=	1.76 pints
1 centimetre	=	0.39 inch (in)

Further reading

Large comprehensive textbooks

Behrman RE, Kleigman RM, Arvin AM (eds). *Nelson Textbook of Paediatrics,* 15th edn. WB Saunders, 2001.

Campbell AGM, McIntosh N (eds). *Forfar and Arneil's Textbook of Pediatrics,* 5th edn. Churchill Livingstone, 1998.

Roberton N.R., Rennie J.M. (eds). *Textbook of Neonatology,* 3rd edn. Churchill Livingstone, 1999.

Index